Jessie's HOUSE OF NEEDLES

A missionary nurse brings faith and healing to the remote highlands of West Papua

John Algate

JAC Publishing
Brisbane, Australia

Cover photo: Jessie Williamson with clinic workers. *The clinic workers came to the hospital to collect their equipment. Two by two they would go in different directions to visit as many villages as possible.'*

Published by JAC Publishing, Brisbane, Australia

Printed by IngramSpark

Contact author at johnalgate55@gmail.com

Cataloguing-in-Publication details are available from the National Library of Australia

www.librariesaustralia.nla.gov.au

ISBN 978-0-9953583-0-0 (Paperback)

ISBN 978-0-9953583-1-7 (e-Book)

I was asked to come to Korupun because they didn't have a medical program. The church needed someone to train their local people to become clinic workers and midwives. When I arrived the people were not very keen about the clinic because they still had their witch doctors and their medicine men. So we started off with maybe half a dozen people in the clinic. Two years later the clinic was full and I was training six clinic workers a year....

When I first came here the death rate for children under two years was 50 per cent. Now it's down to just one or two (every) couple of months.

- Jessie Williamson

John Algate has more than 40 years'
experience in journalism, politics, com-
munications and marketing. Whatever his
day job – news or political reporter, docu-
mentary maker, speech writer or media
advisor – he never lost his love of writing
and the thrill of unearthing a good story.

Contents

Foreword

For the first 11 years of Jessie Williamson's three-and-a-half decades serving as a nurse with World Team mission amid mountain tribes in West Papua, Indonesia, Carol and I were delighted to be her colleagues. Though we worked amid swamp-dwellers far to the south of Jessie's mountain outpost, we met her at least annually in mission gatherings. Beyond that, Jessie helped Dr. Jack Leng deliver our fourth child, our dear little Valerie, in 1975. When I became ill during an admin trip to Karubaga, none other than Jessie diagnosed me with Hepatitis C and ordered me home for six weeks of bedrest!

Now, reading John Algate's *Jessie's House of Needles*, I discover that what we and others saw Jessie accomplishing during her first years at Karubaga was merely a prelude to her exponentially wider ministry in later years. It seemed amazing enough that Jessie *herself*, facing the occasional absence of a doctor at World Team's Karubaga hospital, administered procedures that normally would be performed only by fully trained physicians in hospitals elsewhere.

I refer to procedures such as removing a barbed arrow or spear-tip that is deeply embedded in a patient's back or thigh and then suturing the gash! Or tilting a baby in a mother's womb so that it could then be born head-first rather than foot-first or hand-first! Or, later at Korupun, performing an episiotomy in a cramped tribal hut with naught but a flashlight and a crackling fire to illumine the patient!

What amazed everyone in West Papua even more was to see Jessie begin training hundreds of newly Christian, newly literate tribal youth to perform similarly complex medical procedures on their own. Jessie did this in more and more locations, including for missions other than World Team. She taught trainees to dosage penicillin for pneumonia, sulpha drugs for dysentery, iodine for goiter, chloroquine for malaria and tetracycline for other diseases. She even arranged for Mission Aviation Fellowship (MAF) pilots to resupply her trainees with medicine via airdrops in areas where aircraft could not land.

Many of Jessie's trainees pioneered medical ministry in remote valleys, enabling needy patients to be treated where they lay rather than be carried or struggle on their own over steep, often slippery mountain trails to find help. But if trekking was indeed required because a helicopter was not available or weathered in, Jessie taught her trainees to arrange for a patient to be transported on a stretcher consisting of two poles stuck through the four corners of a 100-kilo rice sack!

Jessie also urged trainees to teach the Gospel of Christ to the people they served. As a result, while adult and especially infant mortality rates were diminishing, additional churches were not only planted but also began to flourish. Long-stagnant population growth rates began to rise even at a distance from outposts where Western missionaries themselves resided.

Not long before her death, Jessie agreed to publication of a book about her life with the proviso that she not be portrayed as an evangelical 'Mother Teresa'. That the Australian government had recognised her with a medal of honor was more than enough! However, I personally believe greater recognition is indeed well merited. Though Jessie might chide me when I meet her in Heaven, still I believe Bible-believing Christians everywhere will do well to recognize Jessie Williamson posthumously as exactly what her proviso dismissed.

Mother Teresa served long and faithfully in urban India where taxis, law enforcement and medical supplies were readily available. Everyone around Mother Teresa spoke or at least understood the same language—Hindi.

Furthermore, Mother Teresa enjoyed support and publicity from the Vatican.

Evangelist-nurse Jessie served about as long and just as faithfully among warring Dani and Kimyal tribal people hidden away amid West Papua's rugged, earthquake-and-landslide-prone mountains. Yet Jessie and her numerous trainees also influenced people in at least 10 other remote outposts as well. In some places, as many as eight languages had to be learned or at least interpreted. Moreover, all the while—with logistic help from her World Team colleagues and MAF—Jessie had to inspire individual backers to support her by maintaining a constant flow of correspondence with friends in her homeland. Excerpts from that poignant correspondence abound in this book.

Jessie Williamson is a godly and ingeniously heroic example of Christlike servanthood. Spread the word, fellow Christians! Urge everyone you know to be blessed and inspired by *Jessie's House of Needles*—an epic biography.

Don Richardson

Author of *Peace Child, Lords of the Earth,* and other books

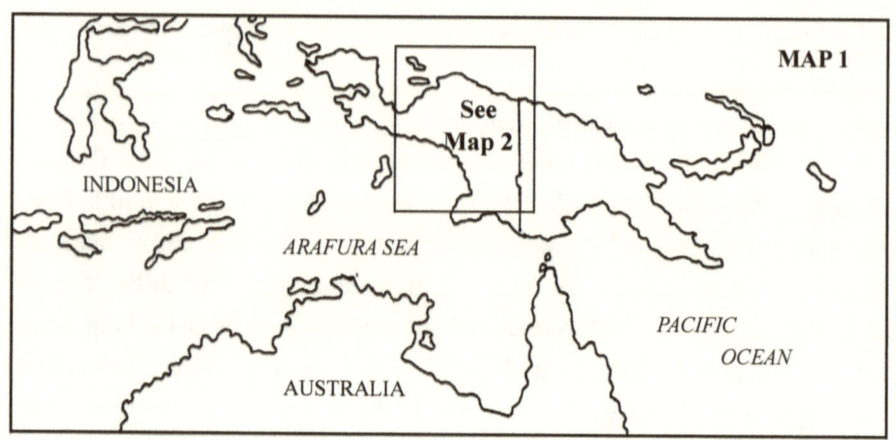

MAP 1
INDONESIA
See
Map 2
ARAFURA SEA
AUSTRALIA
PACIFIC
OCEAN

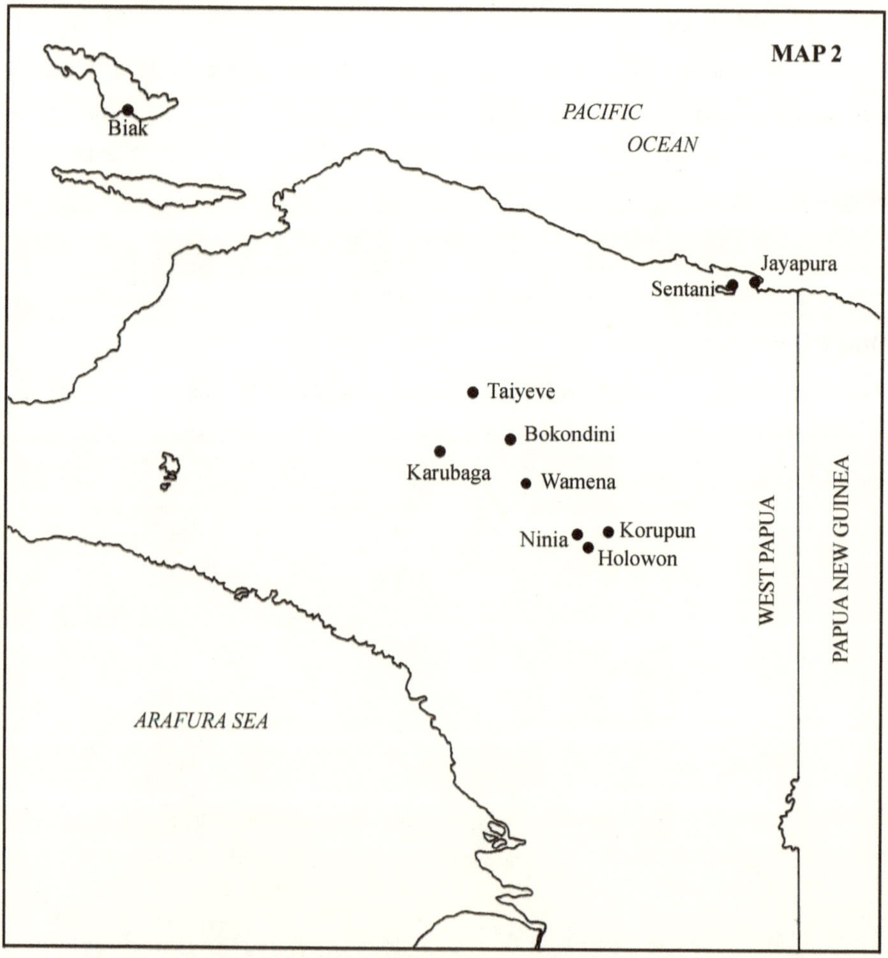

MAP 2
Biak
PACIFIC
OCEAN
Jayapura
Sentani
Taiyeve
Bokondini
Karubaga
Wamena
Ninia
Korupun
Holowon
WEST PAPUA
PAPUA NEW GUINEA
ARAFURA SEA

Introduction

Jessie's House of Needles tells the story of Jessie Williamson, a remarkable Australian who served as a missionary nurse in wild and remote parts of West Papua[1] for 35 years. Jessie toiled tirelessly to improve the health and wellbeing of local people in one of the most untouched, isolated and fascinating corners of the planet. Through faith, commitment, skill, resourcefulness and perseverance she patiently learned local languages, nursed, evangelised and built networks of local medics and midwives who today continue her work among the Dani, Kimyal, and other Indigenous people of West Papua. It is a remarkable legacy that brought Jessie considerable recognition in both her church family, and the broader Australian and international community, including her induction as a Member of the Order of Australia (AM) on Australia Day 1998 for her 'service to international humanitarian assistance'.

Wherever you see italicised text in *Jessie's House of Needles* it is Jessie speaking from the pages of hundreds of prayer letters, private correspondence and other writings that have been preserved by her family. The lively letters not only track her own life and work but also provide eyewitness accounts of droughts, earthquakes, rebel wars, murders and the spiritual

---

1 The administrative arrangements and official names for the western half of the island of New Guinea have changed many times over the years and further changes are mooted at the time of writing. While West Papua is the generic term used in this book, comments that are directly quoted retain the speaker's original words - Irian Jaya, West Irian and so on - to reflect the flavour of the times and their historical context.

and cultural conflicts that came with the encroachment of the outside world on previously closed communities.

Each letter, often hastily drafted at the end of long, demanding days with all the challenges and human dramas involved, was a snapshot in time, capturing both cataclysmic events and touching moments as they unfolded. This posthumous memoir built on edited extracts from Jessie's writings is broadly chronological, but it is also thematic. Because Jessie lived so many years in the highlands her snapshots, when grouped together and placed in context, tell much of West Papua's emergence into the modern world and the central role Christian missionaries played in that process.

Jessie was both a witness and participant in the rapid transformation of the stone-age societies of West Papua with all its triumphs and tragedies, social, religious and political confrontations, life and deaths struggles, earthquakes, droughts, and the uneasy clash of old Gods and new beliefs.

1. First contact... first impressions

The task here is enormous for which I am inadequate, but 'with God all things are possible'.

Jessie Williamson struggled to suppress her excitement as the small Cessna plane of the Mission Aviation Fellowship (MAF) lifted off from Biak Island and turned towards the mainland of West Papua, then known as West Irian. Jessie strained for her first glimpse of this strange new land that would be her home and passion for the next 35 years. It was *a thrill to watch the green shores of West Irian come into sight* she wrote a few weeks later in the first of hundreds, perhaps thousands, of prayer letters to friends and supporters in Australia. Just 27 years of age, Jessie, a missionary nurse, was beginning a fascinating new stage of her life journey. On Saturday, 14 May 1966, she arrived in a dangerous and exciting land to live and work with tribal people. Many were still cannibals who had yet to encounter the outside world, let alone Christian missionaries with their new faith, customs and values.

After touching down at Sentani Airport near the coastal border town of Jayapura Jessie spent a further 10 days cooling her heels while her paperwork was processed. Only then could she fly to the interior and begin her first posting at the remote and isolated Karubaga Station in the Central Highlands. You gain a sense of the personality, humour, enthusiasm and optimism of Jessie Williamson from her first letter home.

Let me bring you up to date since I left Melbourne on 9 May. Arriving in Jakarta at 4.30 pm I was hit by a blast of hot air as I stepped off the plane. This was a signal to hurriedly shed the remainder of my winter clothes.

First impressions…Heat, dust, mosquitoes and hundreds of people everywhere. New sights, smells and tastes….

The years of waiting and anticipation were finally over. Now her training and experience as nurse, midwife and novice missionary would be tested under the most demanding and difficult of circumstances. The bright-eyed optimism that accompanied Jessie's arrival in the highlands would be challenged many times in the years ahead for times were changing fast in West Papua. Sometimes the missionaries worked tirelessly for change, other times they worked equally tirelessly to mitigate against its excesses. If West Papua was all new to Jessie, western medicine, western culture, western religion and western concepts were equally new to the local Dani. It was a big learning curve for everyone.

The people were not used to a hospital. They were frightened and didn't like sleeping in a bed. In the morning I sometimes came in and found them sleeping under the bed and the relatives in the bed. We had one man who nearly burnt the hospital down as he said he couldn't sleep without a fire in his room. Fortunately we found the fire he lit before it did any major damage. So we built a hospital village with 10 little huts. The patients could stay in the huts with their relatives with a fire burning in the centre of each hut. We found that all the people recovered faster and were much happier in a more familiar, village environment.

Our little hospital was kept very busy because at the time it was the only decent hospital in the highlands. MAF would often fly in patients from other areas. We had no roads, no cars and no way to communicate except through two-way radio.

Karubaga enjoyed better flying weather than many villages in the highlands, making it a sensible location for the Regions Beyond Missionary Union's (RBMU – later World Team) base and hospital. By the time Jessie arrived its Christian Leadership Training School had taken firm roots at Karubaga under the astute leadership of West Papuan veteran John Dekker.

The campus included five school buildings, a chapel and two houses for missionaries as well as three hut villages where students would build their own huts when they came to Karubaga to train.

The small Karubaga hospital became the main focus of Jessie's working life for the next 13 years and was an important part of the mission's growing presence in the highlands. Over the previous decade a small band of dedicated evangelists had planted a strong foothold in the Swart Valley. The mission station and its one-doctor hospital was an oasis in a wilderness surrounded by thousands of square kilometres of dense forests and mist shrouded mountains. It was the missionaries, rather than the underfunded and overstretched government in faraway Jakarta that introduced a semblance of modern infrastructure, health and education services to the highlands. Airstrips were few and far between, usually little more than narrow, bumpy, rough-hewn tracks just big enough to take the small planes that provided a lifeline to the highlands. Take-offs and landings were an adventure in themselves and flying could be treacherous in the fast changing weather. Jessie often operated the early morning radio schedule.

This enabled us to find out about weather patterns which dictated when planes could land. We could also let MAF know about emergencies and pass on messages to other members of the mission although we could not speak to them directly.

Other times Jessie talked to the pilots as they approached, because cloud could roll in very quickly and reduce visibility making it impossible to land. Everyone knew that a plane that crashed in the jungle might never be found. It really was life on the edge, even more so in those early years before the government's presence increased and foresters and miners moved in to exploit the region's rich resources.

Any passing illusions young Jessie, or "Nona Yetty" as the Dani called her because of their difficulty pronouncing J and S, may have harboured about the romanticism of mission life in the highlands of West Papua were quickly reined in. There were overwhelming demands for health and medical services in a land sadly lacking in both.

The ambush and spearing of fellow missionary Stan Dale soon after her arrival reinforced the personal dangers and risks faced by missionaries living in this remote wilderness.

2. An eye opening initiation

We treated many accidents… people involved in wars who came in with spears and arrows in different parts of their anatomy, adventurous people falling out of trees and down cliffs.

Life was hectic, and so different from anything Jess had experienced before. Most men wore only a penis gourd and the women skimpy grass skirts. Jessie was always interested in local culture, but, like most outsiders, struggled to comprehend some of its more brutal manifestations. Women often had knuckles cut from their fingers, apparently to appease the spirits following the death of a close relative, and babies were sometimes thrown over waterfalls to ensure protection for their crops and family.

Such was the place Jessie had chosen to be. It was a challenging and dangerous choice. Just 10 days after she touched down at Karubaga station Jessie saw first-hand the personal risks facing her and her colleagues

Jack Leng, (the station doctor) *knocked on my door to tell me there had been a message from Ninia. Pat Dale, wife of missionary Stan Dale, had heard via the Dani villagers that her husband had been killed and the rest of the group ambushed by hostile Yali tribesmen who were now coming to kill Pat and the children. She needed an aeroplane to get out as soon as possible.*

Initially the mission planned to fly Dr Leng into Ninia, just in case Stan had been wounded and not killed, as the Dani word for 'kill' and 'unconscious' can be confused. Jack asked me to organise an emergency box for him to take on the plane. Never having dealt with arrow and spear wounds I was a little confused as to what to pack.

But the weather deteriorated rapidly and plans changed accordingly. Dr Leng was put on hold and the aircraft flew straight to Ninia to pick up Pat Dale and the children and bring them safely to Karubaga. The revised arrangements meant Dr Leng would then take the return flight to Ninia.

Things did not happen as planned. As the plane landed at Ninia to pick up Pat and the children there was a great shout from the people. A group of men carrying a stretcher had just come into view.

Stan was with them, alive and conscious, but suffering numerous arrow wounds that required urgent surgery. So an hour later the plane, carrying Stan, Pat and the children touched down at Karubaga to find a medical team busily preparing for their arrival. Jessie, who had first met Stan when he was a patient at the Alfred Hospital in Melbourne, was one of them.

Stan told us his story. He and some Christian Yali men had gone to investigate a report that two Yali evangelists had been ambushed and killed. They (Stan's small party) were accompanied by an Indonesian policeman. The party walked over the mountains for six hours, arriving at dusk in the Yali village where the murders had occurred. Stan and his party were ambushed. Stan received five arrow wounds and other members of the party were also wounded. The policeman shot off his gun and frightened the hostile villagers away. They then took shelter in a nearby village house that was set aside for visitors. Five arrow wounds would normally result in infection and death. Their situation was serious.

As the men huddled around inside the little house the Yali helpers told Stan: 'We must not stay here the night. The attackers will be back in the morning to kill and eat us.' As soon as the excited village people settled down for the night the group sneaked out of the hut and started off up the mountain. It was raining and the path over the mountain was very steep, narrow and treacherous. Without a light they had to feel their way up and down the mountain paths. After they had been walking several hours Stan told them he couldn't go any further and lay down on the ground. He told the men to go on and leave him. 'No,' they cried, 'We will not leave you. We will carry you.' They cut down saplings to make poles and made a stretcher by lashing the bark from some nearby banana trees around these poles. They placed Stan on the poles, tied him down, and continued on the difficult track over the mountains, arriving back at Ninia at 5.30 the next morning, just in time to be taken out by plane.

Running a hospital in Irian was a little different to running a hospital back home. To start with we had no blood bank and no oxygen. We had to get another doctor from the south coast an hour-and-a-half away. We needed more oxygen and all that was available was the Oxywelding O2 from the MAF. We grabbed people who came in on the planes to check and see if their blood matched with Stan and then sterilised and set up theatre.

Before we started surgery we began to pray. Jack carefully treated all the different wounds that Stan had sustained from the barbed arrows. He had sustained a puncture wound through the chest cavity which should have caused the lungs to collapse. However, when Stan had pulled out the arrow the barbs had pulled out some muscle to plug the hole. He also had another puncture into his abdominal cavity which caused the bowel to be pierced in several places. Eighteen inches of bowel had to be removed. The other wounds were non-invasive and only needed some suturing.

As darkness closed in the small hospital generator fired up to provide light for the surgeons.

It so happened it was one of those nights when the flying ants hatch. Where would they go in their thousands but to the only light in the valley and climb in through the louvre windows? They went straight to the light and then dropped into Stan's abdomen so I spent a lot of time fishing them out.

Jessie was on night duty during the weeks Stan Dale lay ill and in danger of dying.

I would come out of hospital each morning to see the ring of 12 naked men sitting outside. I asked them what they were doing and they said: 'We do not know Stan, but because he came here to tell us about Jesus he is our brother. We know that only the great God can make him better.' This was an encouragement to me, a new missionary, to see their faith. Several years before they had been killing each other.

After six weeks convalescing Stan returned to Ninia and presciently told the villagers: *'Even if I have to die to give the Yali people the Gospel that is OK with me.'*

It was a stimulating and eye opening initiation for the adventurous young Australian starting her nursing ministry. The attack on Stan Dale and his group would have a tragic sequel two years later, one that would reverberate around the world.

3. The house of needles

My clinic now has a new Dani name, the house of needles. Quite appropriate don't you think?

Jessie's letters to family, friends and financial supporters gave regular snapshots of the medical issues that confronted doctors and nurses in Karubaga. It was a big change of pace for anyone new to the mountains, however experienced they may have been in the better resourced hospitals back home.

We get a lot of babies with deformed feet so yesterday I was shown how to put plasters on these, to correct the deformities and give them at least a chance of being able to walk straight. Guess we will have an influx once the word gets round. We haven't had plaster to do it with before. Some has just come in so we will be able to do some until it runs out again. (August 1966)

Medical work has its humorous touches too, as well as its serious ones. One lady came and said that she had been bitten by a pig. Sure enough, her fingers had been bitten off at the first knuckle. Her husband gravely informed me that they had already eaten the pig. Tit for tat! (February 1967)

Now the whooping cough is with us in full force. We were able to do over 1000 vaccinations early in the year when we first heard the epidemic was heading our way. Now the sick ones are those who didn't bother to bring their babies in at that time. These little ones die so fast if not started on injections very quickly. We have had two babies die here. In the area where the epidemic started over 300 babies died in a month.

Just had an interruption – three babies with diarrhoea, one with whooping cough, two with flu. I have lost two already with flu – one day they are O.K. the next they are sick. Deekom (clinic worker) *calls the whooping cough the 'woofing cough'. The closest he could get to it. It sounds funny but I guess a lot of them have real barks anyway.* (August 1967)

Today they brought in a man who was cutting a tree down when it fell on him and fractured his leg. Also a lady whose husband took to her with a piece of firewood that was nicely alight and very hot. So she has an eye injury and a nice big burn down her back and arm which will take a while to heal. (November 1967)

While it took time to adjust to the rigours of the mountains Jessie was a keen learner and took every chance she could to expand her horizons beyond the small hospital and her medical duties.

Over the past few months I have been able to get out to some of the closer churches with some of the other missionaries. About one to one-and-a-half hour's walking. I am certainly getting my 'mountain legs', but still have 'weak legs' as the Dani people put it. The steep mountains clothed in tall trees, waving grasses and swift roaring rivers are a constant reminder that our Creator has made all this wonderland and beauty...

It is such a joy at the end of a hot steep climb to find crowds of eager people waiting for us and joyfully welcoming us into their midst. If it happens to be a weekday they all have a 'stop work meeting' for the day and stay home instead of going to the gardens, so they will be sure not to miss any of the 'living words'. These words they hear they store up in their memories and go out to other villages to tell them. The people listen as they gather around their fires in their little huts in the evening. (May 1967)

Jessie and her colleagues were providing health services to people with little or no understanding of the science that underpinned this new 'magic'.

The Dani folk firmly believe that if the doctor 'cuts them up' it is the cure for all ills. They see things like a boy's hand being made useable again after many years of inactivity due to bad burns as a child. Cutting, suturing and skin grafts and presto four whole fingers again instead of four useless stuck together ones. It takes some explaining why someone with a very large liver and spleen plus ascites cannot be fixed in the same way. (April 1971)

Sitting in a dark little hut with a group of anxious faces surrounding me I thought what a tremendous contrast this was to a hospital situation at home. Helen Dekker called me to say that one of the Bible School women had haemorrhaged and was unconscious. I grabbed my little blue bag and a bottle of intravenous fluid and ran.

As we endeavoured to get the intravenous into a vein that had all but collapsed we were conscious of the Lord's guiding hand. IV in and running well, the patient beginning to come back to life. I glanced round. Husband and relatives all sitting around on the floor, very quiet and serious – the light of the lamp throwing shadows over the faces and the IV quite out of place hanging from the low ceiling by a piece of string. What a joy to be able to help in such a situation. (June 1972)

Reading through Jessie's writings you are struck by the sheer scale of the need and the depth of human tragedy as epidemics swept through the highlands. In 1968 Jessie's account of a flu epidemic graphically brought news of another epidemic to her network and supporters at home.

'Three people in that village have died, two people in that village up there, four in the one across the river and one up on the mountain. That makes this many,' said Deekom, the head clinic worker as he held up both hands. Hong Kong flu was raging around Karubaga. What could we do? The eight clinic workers were frantically busy treating 400 patients each morning at the two clinics. They were tired after a busy day's work but their desire to help their friends and relatives was much stronger.

'Yes' they all said, 'we will go out to the villages and take medicine to those who cannot come in.' Often, because everyone was sick, there was no one available in these villages to carry in the very ill for treatment and so they just died.

The clinic workers came to the hospital at 2 pm to collect their equipment. One bowl to boil up needles and syringes, aspirin, vitamins and penicillin. Two by two they would go in different directions to visit as many villages as possible before dark. Sometimes they stayed out overnight, returning only when their supplies had run out. We had enough medicines on hand to deal with this emergency. Over 50,000 aspirins were used during the epidemic and hundreds of bottles of penicillin. Eighty-three people died around Karubaga. Our stocks are very low now.

Such tragedies were all too common. Time and again over the years Jessie reported on the 'dying' season when epidemics swept the highlands.

'Yetty I have a sore throat, my tongue is sore, my back hurts, my head is hot, I feel sick all over.' Oh dear! The flu has come to stay. We do praise the Lord for the supply of aspirin that we received last week but our penicillin and sulpha tablets are about non-existent. This flu is turning into pneumonia in the older folk and we are in a very desperate situation. I have had penicillin on order for four months but there is none in Jayapura to be had.

'Yetty can I have some aspirin to go out to some of the far villages where the people are too sick to come in and there is no one to carry them.' Clinic workers going the second mile in the afternoons after a very busy morning in the clinic to try to help their friends in the outer areas. Both clinics here on the station have been seeing approximately 200 people each morning. There have been five deaths out in the villages of folk who didn't come in for treatment. This is a hard time for the Dani folk. (March 1974)

I was called to one of the little round huts late one afternoon by one of the clinic workers who was concerned about a baby whose mother had just brought him in. Wrapped in an old piece of calico that had long since come off a parcel, she showed me the wasted figure of a little two-year-old, a desperately sick little baby. That was all the covering it had. No other clothes or blankets and it was a cold night. The sad mother had walked six hours to bring the little one in, but too late. She wailed and wailed for her baby but to no avail. (1976)

The tragedies are compounded by our knowledge that so many of these illnesses were curable, treatable or avoidable if the right medicines, vaccinations or treatments were available. Day in, day out, Jessie and her colleagues did what they could to meet the health needs of Karubaga, saddened by the tragedies, but also celebrating their many successes.

We treat approximately 15,000 people in our small hospital and three clinics in one month. The drugs and money for our work come from interested friends at home. (1975-76)

A day of great rejoicing next week when a boy we have done five skin grafts on will be ready to go home. His people were sure he would die because he was so badly burnt so we praise the Lord we are able to send him back alive. Do pray for this boy from the Sela Valley as he returns to his people. Most are cannibals but there are Dani evangelists in his area and some of his people are listening to the word of God. (March 1976)

We performed an emergency operation immediately on a lady sent in from the South Coast. She was very shocked on arrival with hardly any blood pressure or pulse. First we had to find someone with the same blood type in order to give her a blood transfusion before we could start. Our operating theatre although small, is quite adequate, and the operating table of ancient vintage still works well. Three hours later, weary and hot from the afternoon sun streaming in the windows, we put in the last stitches, not for the tubal pregnancy as we had first thought, but from a ruptured spleen. (April 1977)

A lot of patients flown in from other areas are midwifery problems that missionaries with no medical training are glad to send off to the doctor. Dr Donaldson, our new doctor, said that most of these cases are completely new to him. He had only read about them in books and had never actually seen them in real life. He is surely getting educated quickly....One lady that was flown in had been in labour for seven days. (1976)

The medical needs were always far greater than the capacity of the health services to meet them. Doctors were precious resources and there were never enough, even in the good times, let alone the bad when personal dramas, ill-health, staff shortages or routine leave and furloughs had an impact.

Do pray for the medical needs up here at present. Dr Dresser from The Evangelical Alliance Mission hospital has had to go home on account of his son's serious illness. Dr Wright from the Australian Baptist Mission Society hospital has had his visa cancelled and is now in the process of reapplying. Dr Powell from the Unevangelized Fields Mission Hospital is on restricted activity because of his health. Our doctor is due for furlough in July, which will leave the doctor from the German Mission the only mission doctor available for emergencies for the interior of Irian Jaya. This will be a tremendous load on him and he will need much help and strength from his Lord to cope. (April 1977)

Despite such setbacks Jessie kept plugging away at the never ending demand for medical care, earning the respect of her colleagues as she did so.

Kathryn Kline recalls that Jessie had 'a good level head on her shoulders' and 'was a nurse by gift and talent'.

'Jessie was my mentor as a nurse and midwife; she could do all that I wished I could do, and I learned many things about nursing from her. Jessie is very caring, and very capable with patients. I worked with Jessie at the Karubaga clinic and hospital as an assistant. She was well trained and experienced and knew what to do in difficult medical situations.'

4. Finding God and nursing

We went to church once a fortnight when there was a minister available. I never dreamt of becoming a missionary. In fact I didn't know what a missionary did.

Karubaga and the missionary life was a world apart from Jessie's roots in a small farming community in Australia. Born into a dairying family on 4 November 1938, Jessie was the ninth of 10 children. She was christened Roseabel Jessie Williamson but always called Jessie because, as sister Thelma explained in Jessie's eulogy:

'An enthusiastic father registering his baby daughter forgot the order of the names. As this was then a legal document Jess went through life explaining her first name.'

The children were raised on a small farm at a place called Greenvale, now a suburb of Melbourne but then quite an isolated little farming community. It was, as Thelma recalls, a frugal, rustic but carefree existence reminiscent of the experiences of other small farm families of the time.

'The last three of our family, Jessie, Pam and myself, were known as 'the kids' and we were harum scarum little country kids. We rode the farm horse three or four up at a time. We all had our farm chores. Our parents, Bertha Zerbe of German descent and Hugh with Scottish forebears were wonderful role models of courage and strength in adversity, through drought and financially hard times. We all learned the value of the 'work ethic', honesty and integrity. Our Mother took us to the tiny Methodist church whenever there was a visiting pastor. We had no electricity until we were in our teens. We lived with kerosene lanterns; a Tilley lamp sat on our dining room table; we carried candles to move around the house and we had a fuel stove.'

Jessie's father never learned to drive a car so the family travelled around the district by horse and jinker. Even today there are local reminders of Jessie's pioneering forebears with Williamson's Road and Zerbe Reserve preserving the families' association with the Doncaster and Templestowe areas. Thelma has a clear if, like many people looking back, somewhat rosy recollection of family life during those austere war years, including one of Jessie's early dices with danger.

'On New Year's Day we would travel from Greenvale across to Doncaster to visit relatives who had an orchard. We would receive boxes of summer fruits to take home for our mother to make into preserves and jam. We remember having very stiff little legs from being squeezed into the front of the jinker for hours. Dad did all the farm work with a team of draught horses. At the end of the day we would go down the paddock to meet him as he unharnessed the horses, they would then come up to the stable to be fed, still with the big harness collars around their necks. We loved him to throw us up on the horse's back behind the harness collar where we would really enjoy the ride home. We would have been four or five years old. I have a vivid memory of one day Jessie's horse deciding to go for a drink in the dam first. As he went down the steep bank, poor little Jessie slid down his neck with the big collar and was perched precariously behind the horse's ears, inches from deep water. Dad followed in hot pursuit and all was well, one frightened little girl and a story we have never forgotten.'

Like all the Williamson children Jessie attended the Greenvale Primary School, a one room school where each class had their own row of desks.

There was one teacher and always around 20 pupils. The older members of the Williamson family, Olive, born in 1921, James, Marjorie, Jean, Joyce and Gordon, didn't have the opportunity for a secondary education, because of a lack of transport.

The next born, Vera, was the first to attend Essendon High School following a government initiative to provide a country school bus service, but left after just one year to work at the local Post Office. Thelma, Jessie and Pamela, the last born in 1941, all attended Essendon High School for four years to gain an Intermediate Certificate.

A little surprisingly it was through school, not church, that Jessie's interest in Christianity developed. She later wrote of her personal 'road to Damascus' experience.

We went to high school by bus. At high school I joined the Inter School Christian Fellowship, (run by Stella Lesley, who remained a lifelong friend, mentor and supporter). *For the first time I was told that the Bible said I was a sinner. I was not too impressed as I always thought that if I went to church and didn't kill anyone - that was all that God expected from me.*

One day as I was coming home from school it was as if God said to me: 'Jessie you have been sitting on the fence for too long [me?]. You have to either accept me or reject me.' That night I knelt by my bedside and asked Jesus to come into my heart and forgive my sin and I wanted to become part of his family. Then I knew that I belonged to Him and He had a plan and purpose for my life as He does for each one of us. Not long after that decision my father had a heart attack and passed away. We had to sell the farm and moved into the city.

Hugh Williamson was just 56 years when he passed away on 7 August 1953 and the family moved to the Melbourne suburb of Essendon. Three years later, on 15 May 1956, Bertha, also aged 56, died of aplastic anaemia, an illness similar to leukaemia that was caused through medical neglect – a failure to check on a side effect of a new antibiotic.

After finishing school Jess worked for a short time in a legal firm until she was old enough to go nursing. She was, from all accounts, an excellent nurse. She won a 'surgical prize' at Footscray District Hospital, now known as Western Hospital Footscray. She gained her second certificate in midwifery at The Queen Victoria Hospital, followed by a third certificate in infant welfare and finally a short course in dentistry. Thus she was highly qualified, particularly for the time.

I had always wanted to become a nurse but because I have a hearing disability I thought it would never happen, however the Lord overruled and I was able to get my general training and midwifery.

Jessie's hearing problems probably began when she was about eight years of age. Thelma recalls a specific childhood incident which Jessie believed triggered the hearing loss.

'We were up in a pepper tree playing horses with an old saddle when we decided to have stirrups and attached some old metal stirrups to a rope and threw it over the branch. Jess put her foot in the stirrup to swing up over the saddle but of course with nothing to anchor it the other stirrup flew back over the branch with great force and whacked her in her ear. I think her hearing loss was gradual but certainly all her adult life she was totally deaf in that ear. She did seek specialist opinions but it appears there was never anything they could do to help. It was a miracle they ever accepted her to do nursing. She never had any sort of hearing aid. I am sure Jess would have had difficulty at times hearing in a nursing class situation, using a stethoscope and the like. She was very determined, although at times a little hesitant to ask you to repeat something if she couldn't hear.'

Jessie grew up in a rustic but loving home. While there was a world of difference between the farm life of her childhood in Australia and the third world realities of life in the remote highlands of West Papua, Thelma astutely observes that there were also some unexpected links between Jessie's two worlds.

'Looking back on Jessie's childhood she was in many ways well acquainted with what would be required of her in later years in a more primitive setting. Not many girls would be unfazed at having to pack a fuel stove onto a ship as part of her job requirements and what's more, know how to use it.'

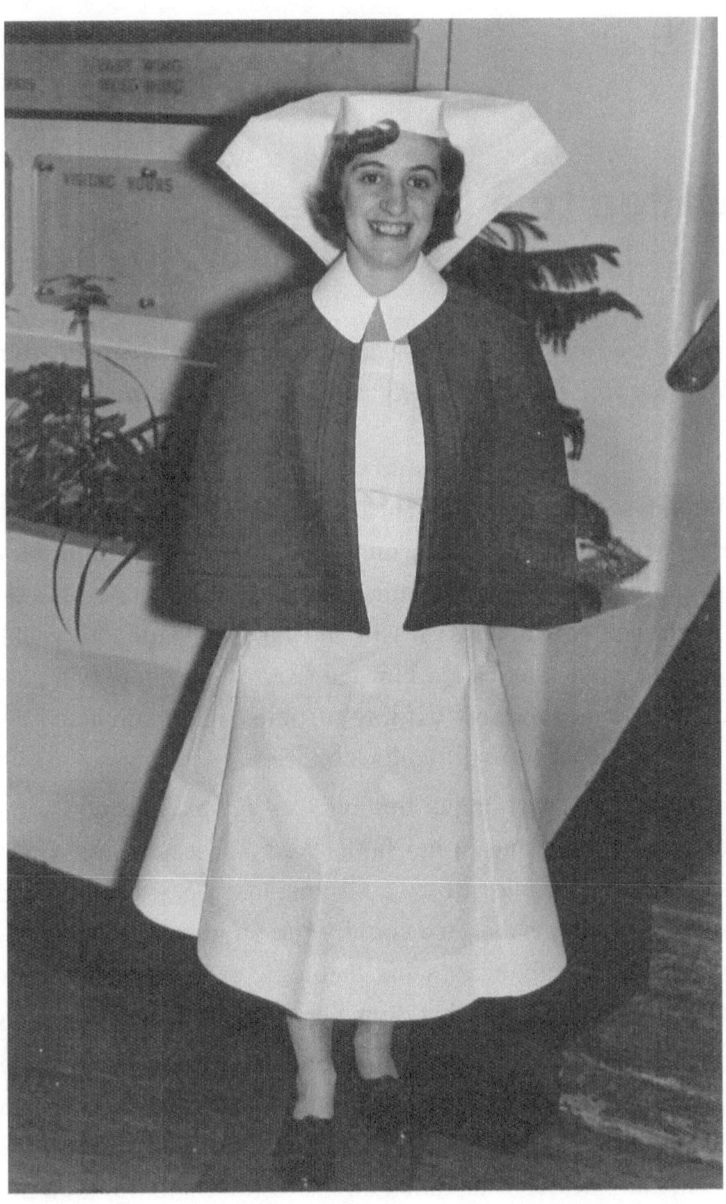

5. Called to a hard life

I felt missionaries needed to be special people with all kinds of gifting and I couldn't even sing in tune. I felt far too inadequate for that kind of work.

Jessie Williamson was an evangelical Christian. She firmly believed that God called her to be a missionary nurse and do his work among stone-age tribal people in West Papua, a dangerous and inhospitable place. Where others might see coincidence, Jessie and her colleagues invariably saw God's guiding hand. She called him the *God of the Impossible*, accepted his wisdom even at the most baffling of times, and maintained her faith through all the dangers and difficulties of life.

It wasn't that she was unquestioning – all people question sometimes – but she was unwavering in her faith. We could easily edit God out of Jessie's memoirs. It would still be a fascinating story – but it wouldn't be Jessie's story any more than we could write an honest account of Albert Schweizer without reference to his theology, or Mother Teresa without understanding her faith and what drew her to the back streets of Calcutta.

All mainstream Christian denominations believe the Bible is the word of God, setting out God's blueprint for how we should live our lives and how Christians should express and share their faith. Jesus is seen also as a great teacher and healer who called on his followers to do likewise, serve the poor, heal the sick and spread God's message throughout the world so all could be 'saved' and have eternal life. Thus believers who devote their lives to Christian endeavour often talk of being called to service. This call can be very personal – God to them. It is God's call and God's decision, no matter how difficult, inconvenient or illogical that decision may appear at the time.

In her later years Jessie recounted her call to missionary service and how she felt 'challenged' to attend Bible College. She was in her mid-twenties and had worked hard to become a nurse. Despite the 'challenge' she was tired of study and reluctant to begin another demanding course. As so often happened in her life, inspiration came from the Bible, this time from 2 Timothy 2:15: *study to show yourself approved unto God, a workman that needeth not be ashamed, rightly dividing the word of truth.*

Overcoming her earlier misgivings Jessie enrolled in a two-year course at the Melbourne Bible Institute in 1963. The College was founded in 1920 specifically to train missionaries to serve with the China Inland Mission. Its founder was a colourful, intelligent, capable, but occasionally wayward former Anglican cleric, Reverend Clifford Nash. Still, he left a significant legacy because the Institute he founded, now known as the Melbourne School of Theology, has since trained some 5000 missionaries, including Jessie.

As I got near the end of my training I was praying that the Lord would show me what next!! I was challenged about going overseas but I said no way Lord I am too ordinary. I felt far too inadequate for that kind of work.

Despite such personal misgivings Jess applied to RBMU to work in Indonesia.

The mission accepted me but said that Indonesia at that time was a closed country as they had not been able to get a visa for four years.

Jessie could be head strong, particularly when she found Biblical inspiration to support her view. She felt called to serve in Indonesia and found scriptural solace for her determined stance in a verse from Revelations 3 that says: *'I have set before you an open door and no man can close it.' I needed that encouragement. As time went on people kept saying that they thought I had my wires crossed because it was taking so long and I should go to Africa.*

But Jessie was patient. Instead of rushing into an alternative posting she spent her time building skills she would need later in West Papua.

Some friends said to me: 'Jessie, if you are going to a third world country you should be able to pull teeth.' Ugh. I applied to the Dental Hospital for a short course in pulling teeth. If you came to the Dental Hospital at that time you could have had your tooth pulled by Jessie for 20 cents.

During her last term of training Jessie shared a bedroom with Norma Stephenson who became another life-long friend and supporter. Norma recalls the final term as something of a blur with final exams looming and all the normal busyness of young lives.

It isn't clear how Jessie supported herself during her two full-time years of study, or in the period after she completed her study and awaited her first posting. No one in the family was in a position to offer much financial support during those years and her siblings assume she supported herself from her savings and by occasional relief work as a nurse, a practice she continued in later years to supplement her missionary stipend. Thelma recalls that:

> 'Sometimes when Jessie was home on furlough (from West Papua) and needed some cash she would fill in for the matron at Gisborne Hospital who was delighted to find someone who could cope with what was known as a 'bush hospital'. This allowed her to go on holiday.'

Jess's sisters, Marj Bradley and Joyce Taylor lived in Gisborne, 55 kilometres north-west of Melbourne, and would have known the matron of the Hospital, so Jessie may have also worked there during the long delay between Bible College and her posting to Indonesia.

> 'Mention of Gisborne rang a very faint bell somewhere *way* at the back of my mind, so she might well have been working there until her visa was through,' suggested Norma Stephenson who had moved to Adelaide soon after graduating from Bible College.

'When I was in Adelaide, we were in constant mail contact and I used the money I earned buying clothes etc. for Jessie's 'kit'. I had all her sizes with me, and I can assure you, the sizes for assorted garments I purchased, were somewhat different from what she would have worn later on. But we were all skinny in those days!'

As for Jessie:

Time was marching along and again people were wondering about my visa. We had applied but things go slowly in Indonesia. The first lot of application papers were lost in the mail and then after we had sent the next lot we got a letter from our Jakarta office to say not to apply for any more visas because it was causing trouble for them with the immigration office. Then on the same day, written by the same man we received a letter saying, 'Tell Jessie to go ahead with her application'. Wow. The Lord wonderfully gave me a visa much to the amazement of everybody except God.

More earthly forces may also have been in play. It is estimated that more than 500,000 Indonesians were slaughtered in brutal reprisals following a failed communist coup on 30 September 1965. Most of those massacred were Abangan Muslim communists. The Abangan faith mixed Islam with other religions and religious practices and following the coup, many Abangans were pressured to dissociate themselves from communism by converting to other religions like Hinduism and Christianity so Christianity was again, if only temporarily, in favour in Indonesia.

This is consistent with Norma Stephenson's recollection of the times. She recalls that the 'door to Indonesia was closed until after the Communist coup. Once that was dealt with by the government, they opened the door to Christian missions in an attempt to prevent further spread of communism's influence.'

Whatever the cause, the visa approval, the good news Jess had long anticipated and planned for, had finally come through and her missionary adventure could begin.

6. Mission Aviation Fellowship (MAF)

Calling Karubaga – Calling Karubaga. This is the way our day begins when the MAF radio call comes through at 7 am each day.

Trekking and moving goods and supplies from the coast to the highlands was a near impossible task. There were no roads and barely a network of useable tracks to move from one village to another or one valley to the next. There were no modern settlements, supply routes or supply chains to support the pioneering missionaries; just kilometre after kilometre of crocodile and snake infested malarial swamp with a near impenetrable barrier of tangled jungle and rainforest and that was before you reached the wet, windy, wild and treacherous mountain slopes with their seemingly endless lines of knife-edge ridges and ravines.

No wonder then that the first evangelists from the Christian and Missionary Alliance (C&MA) looked to the sky to help establish their first base in the highlands. On April 20 1954 the mission's Irish-built amphibious aircraft, *The Gospel Messenger*, lifted off from the Paniai Lakes area. It flew due east with seven people on board. A couple of hours later *The Gospel Messenger* landed on a wide stretch of the Baliem River and its passengers disembarked to set up camp and live out a long-held dream of bringing Christianity to the mountains.

Soon a series of regular flights were bringing more mission workers and supplies to the valley. In its first year *The Gospel Messenger* made more than 160 round trips to the Baliem Valley, carried more than 200 passengers and delivered 175,000 pounds (80,000 kilos) of equipment and supplies. It was a precious lifeline which set the benchmark for future operations.

Flying in the highlands was demanding and dangerous work. Just how dangerous became all too clear on 29 April 1955 when word came through that pioneering pilot Al Lewis and *The Gospel Messenger* had gone missing in remote country during a routine flight. Twenty-nine days passed before the plane's wreckage was spotted on a ridge east of the Baliem Pass though it would be a further four years before a ground party finally reached the crash site, found and buried the aviator's remains.

While the C&MA immediately ordered a new 180 Cessna the days of individual missions providing their own airplanes was near an end. That role was soon taken over by the the specialist MAF, a joint Australia-U.S. operation which had begun flying out of Madang in 1951 to service missionaries in the Australian mandated Territory of Papua and New Guinea. In 1955 they expanded into West Papua where they continue to serve evangelical missions operating in the province. Thus it was the MAF that first flew Jessie Williamson to join her fellow RBMU missionaries at her new home at Karubaga in May 1966.

Fans of the popular 1970's television series M.A.S.H. would recall how the sound of a distant chopper would trigger urgent activity at the surgical hospital. Similar scenes were regularly played out in Karubaga.

Suddenly, a drone from the sky. Looking up we can see the flash of the wings of the Cessna coming to land. Unscheduled flight. Who can it be? All sorts of things go through one's mind, but uppermost – a medical emergency. Waiting at the airstrip to greet the Cessna is Dr. Jack Leng. 'Yes Jessie – theatre ready as soon as possible please.' (August 1966)

The whirring of a plane overhead can very quickly dispel the very best laid plans for an afternoon. Just yesterday, one pilot brought in a plane load of patients from an area where they have been fighting. Another pilot called up to say he was at a station and a man had broken his arm, would he bring him in? Yet another pilot called to say he couldn't get through because of bad weather and had on board a missionary's child who had fallen from a tree and broken his arm. No ambulances or police siren to sound a warning but a busy two-way radio is a good substitute. (January 1968)

Flying the highlands with its strong winds, variable weather, dense forests and rugged landscapes was always a dangerous occupation.

'Naltja calling Sentani. Naltja calling Sentani' was the call we heard one Saturday afternoon. MAF Cessna MPK called to say he would be here in 10 minutes and that was half-an-hour ago. This call triggered a full scale search by MAF personnel to try and locate the missing aircraft. Hampered by bad weather for two days very little was accomplished. On the third day a man ran into an outstation and reported that a plane had crashed two-day's walk away. With the help of two helicopters from a nearby mining company the plane was soon found. The pilot had been killed on impact. He had apparently run into bad weather, the clouds had settled around him and he couldn't see where he was going.

Do continue to pray for the MAF pilots as the weather pattern changes so rapidly and they are often in dangerous situations. MAF is our only life line to the outside world from the interior. (July 1971)

The network of airstrips built under mission guidance and employing large teams of local labourers was forever expanding.

This last week there has been much rejoicing in the Holowon Valley as the long awaited day 'arrived' for the opening of the new airstrip. The plane landed without any problems and this will now save the people waiting so long for visits. It takes a full day to trek from Ninia to Holowon and about five to 10 minutes by plane. (February 1972)

Later in the year Jessie reported an unexpected backlash from the single minded focus on building the new airstrip.

Just this last week Bruno de Leeuw and John Wilson flew into the new airstrip. They were very much upset to find that the people there were hungry and without a good supply of potatoes. The reason they gave was that they had worked so hard and so long on the airstrip that they hadn't planted their gardens when they should have done so. Those not interested in listening to the Gospel were blaming the coming of the Gospel for the famine. Bruno is planning to send in some rice to help them. (October 1972)

Supporting the MAF was one of the many non-medical duties that fell Jessie's way as roles and responsibilities changed over time.

My new responsibilities are varied and time consuming. I now have the two-way radio in my house and this often necessitates me being 'on the air' at 5.30 or 6 am with weather reports for the pilots, on at 7 am for the MAF roll call, meeting all planes, checking the load and seeing it off again.

As we (Karubaga) are one of the few stations which usually has reasonable weather most of the time the pilots often use this as an alternative if they can't reach their destination. They often just 'drop in' to sit and wait until the weather clears elsewhere. Tonight we have a pilot weathered in because he couldn't make it back to Sentani through the bad weather. He will be off as soon as it is light at 5.15 am in the morning. (June 1972)

Although medical evacuations saved many lives they were not without their complications.

Just recently a station many miles away called up on the two-way radio to say a man had been hit by a large falling rock. He needed urgent medical attention - could they get some help. He had been carried into the station on an improvised stretcher made from two small trees with vine slung across them. Not a very comfortable trip for a man in agony. On reaching the station, they called for help and very soon a MAF pilot was heading towards Tangma.

On arrival the pilot discovered that the relatives had decided that maybe he shouldn't go after all, in case we used witchcraft at the hospital. After glancing at the patient, the pilot decided that he would die if he wasn't given medical help immediately. With this in mind he argued with the relatives and explained that the personnel at the hospital wanted to help them, not practice sorcery on their friend.

After much talk the pilot took off with the patient and two relatives on board. Because of the delay in leaving it was now getting late and the light was rapidly fading. With the disappearance of the sun we lit huge bonfires along the sides and at the top and bottom of the strip to guide the little Cessna in to land. The operation began and three-and-a-half hours and a few dozen sutures later the patient was taken to one of the little huts adjoining the hospital - much more alive. The damage was extensive and the pilot's estimation of the injury was correct. He would have died without help. Today he is up walking around with the aid of a stick and his face one huge smile. No sorcerer witchcraft involved. Just a team of Christian workers wanting to show the love of God through their skill. (1976)

The small mission hospital had limited resources and sometimes MAF pilots found themselves in the middle of the medical emergency, not just on the periphery flying planes.

What are one of the things a MAF pilot dislikes intensely? What would you think? Yes, someone having a baby in the plane when they are in the air and there is no hostess to take care of the emergency. Usually a frantic call from the air – 'She's having it up here! What do I do?' This has happened to our pilots twice in the past couple of weeks. (1976)

I have taught the pilots how to give injections as I cannot always go along on all the shuttles. They weren't too keen to start, but as they have seen results of their help in this way they have realised how important it is to the local people on the outposts. I have made a little pack to carry in each plane (penicillin and syringe) and they take them wherever they go. One day Bill (a MAF pilot) came and said he had given an injection to a man whose foot was half eaten away and he could even see all the bones exposed. (March 1979)

Clouds were the pilot's great enemy, but even cloudless skies could, in the midst of drought, bring problems.

Our dry season which usually lasts for three weeks has lingered for three months. Because of the very dry weather the people are very busy burning off garden areas. In some places bush fires are raging out of control. The smoke haze has made it difficult and dangerous for the pilots. Some have had to be grounded because of poor visibility. It has to be at least three miles. Pressures begin to build up as they try and crowd too much into the good flying days. They have lost four planes over the past year. (October 1982)

I came back Friday from my week at Sela Valley. The weather has been terrible for this time of year. It was very foggy and it took us 45 minutes to get there instead of the usual 10 minutes as the pilot got lost and we were in the wrong valley. We then had to do a lot of twisting, turning and spiralling to get out. It was like going up a fast lift. I was sure that we would be plastered on the mountainside. I was glad to get out on the ground. Our guardian angels were sure working overtime. (March 1985)

Jessie was in Soba for three days in April 1984 for a mini conference with all 12 missionaries from the Eastern Highland stations.

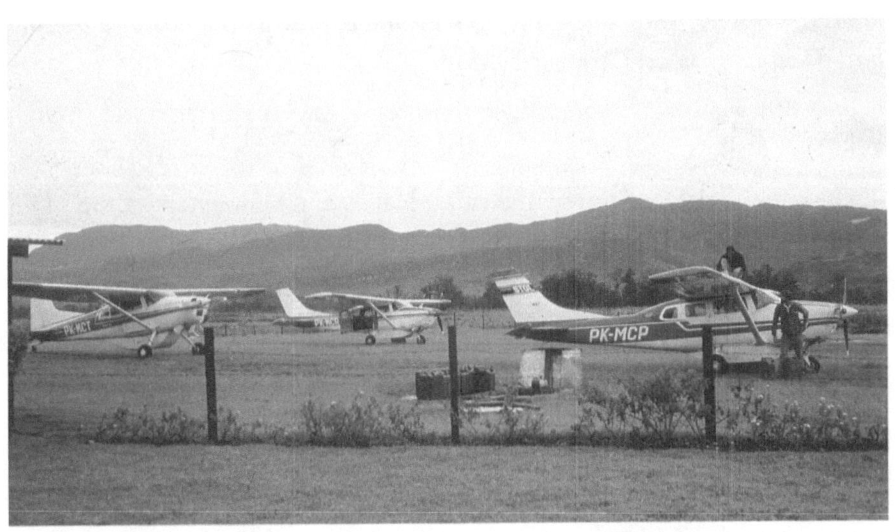

The second day we were saddened to hear that one of the MAF planes had crashed on take-off in Wamena. The pilot has had bad injuries both internal and to the head. The passengers were better off. One had a broken leg and one cuts, and the other had nothing at all which was a miracle. They have asked for nurses to go and help with his nursing care. They have two nurses on day and two on night duty, so that means a lot of people.

In a later letter she provided an update.

The pilot badly injured in the crash has been evacuated to an intensive care unit in Townsville. The latest we have heard is that he is starting to wake up but he has a shattered hip which is going to be a real problem to fix. The two lots of parents have come out to be with him in Townsville. (June 1984)

MAF wasn't the only air operator in West Papua. Both government and private airlines flew commuter planes to the large airstrips like Wamena.

Yesterday we were shocked when we heard that an Indonesian plane had crashed at an interior station because of fog. It had 20 passengers on board. Fortunately it was a mission station where there was a doctor and hospital. Three people died and the rest were injured – four bad with injuries, spinal etc. They flew in a government doctor and operated on the injured. I am not sure where they put all the people as the hospital doesn't have that many beds. (August 1985)

Just this week a Catholic plane went down and is still missing. (March 1986)

Despite the risks of flying, the small planes and helicopters of the MAF were always a vital part of the mission's efforts to deliver services throughout West Papua. Jessie was no exception and spent countless hours making short hops around the mountain villages.

This past week I went by helicopter to another valley to do DPT (triple antigen) vaccinations. The first time ever for these people. I went to three villages and did 250 children so it was a hectic morning. At the last village they were preparing a feast but the pilot said that unless I planned to stay the night we would have to leave because the weather was deteriorating. We all got strapped in and down came the fog! We sat and waited and waited and wondered if we would be able to sneak between the trees and the fog. I was glad to get home that day as I had not gone prepared to spend the night. Shortly after I returned to Korupun the fog moved in so I was glad the helicopter had got away before it settled in for the afternoon. (September 1986)

Several weeks ago we were all shocked when we heard the MAF Twin Otter plane had crashed, killing a very experienced pilot and seven passengers on landing at one of the interior airstrips. He was circling to come in to land when he crashed and it is still uncertain why he crashed. We have a lot of new pilots who are just learning the ropes. Our foggy season is just beginning and this is always a hard time as the weather is so changeable. (June 1987)

Aviation was a high priority and MAF mechanics and pilots needed a diverse set of skills to keep planes flying, and surprisingly, so did Jessie.

I didn't expect to be spending Saturday afternoon putting a patch on the windsock, but I did. The high winds had blown the pole down, bending the frame and so out came my trusty old treadle sewing machine. I was glad it would sew the heavy material. We had a pilot and his wife and family for the weekend, so he kindly put the frame back together for me and the windsock is now flying gaily in the breeze. (February 1990)

In March Sue (Trenier) *and I went across to the Sela Valley to celebrate the reopening and dedication of the new airstrip. It is more then two years since the big landslide demolished the mission houses and covered the air-strip with tons of mud.*

The people have worked tirelessly by themselves to clear the rubble and mud. They have done an excellent job. When we landed there were hun-dreds of excited people lining the sides of the airstrip. When we stopped at the end of the runway, swarms of people surrounded the plane, and hugged and greeted us. Two groups of people detached themselves from the crowd. They were dressed up in their feathers and nose bones. They began to sing and dance around the plane. We were taken to an area they had set up especially for the occasion and had put up benches under the tarpaulin (to keep off the sun and rain) for us to sit on during the proceedings. When all the speeches etc. were finished they had a ceremony of cutting the ribbon to reopen the airstrip. The ribbon, Kimyal style, was a long piece of green bark stretched across the airstrip, which they proceeded to cut with a long bush knife instead of scissors. (June 1993)

Several weeks ago there was another celebration in the Dagi Valley which is a nine-hour walk from Korupun. The people have been working hard on rebuilding the airstrip there for the past 12 months. It was finally approved by MAF and the first landing safely passed. They had planned a big feast with government officials coming in for the dedication. Unfortunately the weather did not cooperate. They had already killed the pigs before they realised the plane couldn't land because of the fog. They had the feast without the special guests. The actual ceremony was held the next day when the weather cleared. (August 1995)

Danger was an ever present fact of life for pilots and while villagers worked hard to keep their airstrips open, the pilots struggled just as hard to keep planes in the air.

Please pray for the MAF as their planes had several incidents in the past month which could have been fatal - one when his engine blew up but was able to land in a small clearing in the jungle; another, when he lost power on take-off; another, when the brakes couldn't hold on a wet strip; and yet another, when he lost power trying to cross a high mountain range. MAF is our lifeline and they need your prayer and support. (August 1993)

Just two weeks ago one of the MAF planes gave a mayday call when he had engine failure. He was high above the clouds so he couldn't see anything until he broke through the overcast and by then he was close to the jungle with nowhere to land, He thought he saw a glint of water out of the corner of his eye so he banked sharply and there in front of him was a straight stretch of water, the only straight stretch for miles in that winding river. He landed safely in the river. Because of the dry spell the river was only three feet deep instead of the usual six feet, and it had a sandy bottom. A real miracle. (September 1996)

Last week we all got a shock when we heard the MAF helicopter 'fell out of the sky' from 50 feet. We are praising the Lord that neither of the two pilots were injured but the helicopter is very ill indeed and may not recover! It rolled as it landed. This has added extra strain on MAF resources for relief flying. (January 1998)

The missions were a small, tight-knit group. Even after Jessie returned to Australia she was kept up to date with their activities, including moments of shared sadness.

Six weeks ago we were all saddened to hear that one of the Heli Mission helicopters (Swiss Mission) was missing in bad weather. He was subsequently found to have crashed into a deep ravine near Soba, which is one of the airstrips in the Eastern Highlands. This has had a tremendous impact on the whole mission family up there as they are such a close knit community and rely on, and care for each other. Neil Roesler, the pilot, had grown up in Irian Jaya as a Mission Kid and it was his dream to one day go back and fly to help the missionaries continue their work. Sadly that only happened four months before the accident. This is the first fatal accident they have had in 10 years and it has affected all the pilots and their wives as well as the missionaries. (November 2004)

It was indeed a small, close and very personal network of mission people. Helicopter mechanic/engineer, Joel Henson, was the first on the scene and was lowered to the crash site from the helicopter. It was his job to inspect the site and take the initial photographs of the crash. Joel had grown up with Neil at Sentani International School and was devastated by Neil's death, as were the many Mission Kids around the world who had been influenced by Neil's life. Such were the close bonds that developed between the small teams of expatriate missionaries and their families.

7. Missions in West Papua

This past month has seen us farewell five Dani teacher/evangelists plus one clinic worker who are now in the Sela Valley. Do pray for these workers as they learn the language and get close to the people. (March 1974)

Portuguese sailors first sighted the coast of West Papua in 1511. Later Spanish, English and Dutch adventurers also showed interest though not enough to colonise this inhospitable land with its malarial swamps, fierce local tribes and no obvious commercial opportunities. In 1828 the Dutch finally claimed sovereignty but were reluctant to take administrative responsibility for the land they claimed. Instead, in 1855 it was Christian missionaries who made the first serious moves to engage with people, hoping to harvest souls where their governments had refused to plant the seeds of settlement. They arrived on the north coast, enjoying modest success converting locals to Christianity, but their reach was limited to the coastal fringes. It wasn't until 1938 that C&MA finally obtained permission to spread the Gospel to the interior and a year later established its first inland base at Enarotali in the Paniai Lakes area. Soon after, World War II intervened, forcing the mission to abandon its evangelising work and flee ahead of the advancing Japanese.

With war ended the missionaries regrouped and returned to West Papua, eager to extend their reach further and further afield. But the Dutch

Government remained reluctant to allow such expansion into areas where they had no administrative control or power to protect the advancing missionaries.

The missions' eyes were set on the Baliem Valley in the Central Highlands but without official approval they could only make occasional excursions to look - but not walk - into the valley nor communicate with the Dani people living there. That changed suddenly in late 1952 when the ban was lifted although it wasn't until May 1953 that the local governor also gave his consent. The Baliem Valley was still marked 'uncontrolled' on Dutch maps and the government made it patently clear it was not responsible for the missionaries or their safety and they would enter at their own risk – which they did.

When *The Gospel Messenger* and its human cargo made the first significant contact with the Dani people by outsiders, it started something of a gold rush among the evangelical protestant missions. Of course, the rich rewards they sought were 'unreached' converts, not mineral wealth.

In *Peace Child* Don Richardson describes the scene in 1955 as Ebenezer G. Vine, the elderly secretary of the Philadelphia Council of the RBMU, rose to address the student body of the Prairie Bible Institute in Alberta Canada. Mr Vine informed the packed auditorium of the RMBU's decision to enter this last great frontier for Christian outreach and laid out the challenge confronting them:

> 'You may be called upon to make the first advance into the midst of entire tribes that have never known any kind of government control, where people are a law unto themselves and where savagery is a way of life…You will encounter customs and beliefs which will baffle you, but which must be understood if you are to succeed.'

Mr Vine's message touched a chord with many of those present including Don and his wife Carol, John Dekker, Phil and Phyllis Masters and a young Winnie Frost, all of whom were later to become friends and colleagues of Jessie and share many adventures, triumphs and tragedies with her.

While each of the Protestant missions was independent, they eagerly cooperated in this exciting and dangerous venture. Three of them, the Australia-Pacific Christian Mission (APCM), the Australian Baptist Missionary Society (ABMS) and the RMBU formed a team to establish a new joint-base on Lake Archbold to act as their beachhead. RMBU was assigned the Swart Valley and established its first mission station at Karubaga in 1957. In *Torches of Joy,* John Dekker writes of "the unique teamwork among the nine evangelical missions comprising 'The Mission Fellowship'." He elaborated:

> 'The Mission Fellowship had 180 western couples and single missionaries working at 40 mission stations scattered throughout the interior and coastal regions. Each mission concentrated its efforts in a given area, avoiding competition or overlapping, and cooperated in opening new areas in Bible translation… The missions joined hands in developing a Bible vocational school and shared personnel as needs arose – a school nurse, a book keeper, a cook for the annual conference.'

Jessie was a multi-skilled missionary nurse who included cooking among her many talents and may have been one of the cooks John Dekker was referring to.

I went out to help cook at the Baptist/APCM conference. We fed between 60 to 75 people each meal, so it kept us hopping. Then on the last day we had a wedding to cater for two APCM missionaries who were to be married. Julie, the other cook, decorated the cake and it looked lovely. Our icing sugar up here always comes like a solid brick. We have to pound it first with a rock, then with a rolling pin and finally with a sieve. It is quite a process. One of the assistants who was helping us in the kitchen was working on this for us. Somehow in the several days it took to get it to a place of being useable some salt got mixed up with the icing sugar. It was the same consistency. The cake looked beautiful but it was awful. Poor Julie felt terrible, but the bride never noticed. A good reminder to us to be sweet all through, not just on the outside. (August 1991)

The Roman Catholic Church was also active in West Papua – often in direct competition with the evangelical missions. Though much of the time the relationship was courteous, tensions would flare on occasions and Jessie did voice some concerns about Catholic theology and rivalry.

'We want a missionary. We want someone to teach us,' has been the plea of the people around Soba, near Ninia, for the last few months. Now, because we have no one to fill their desire they have walked to Wamena, the nearest government station, to ask the Catholic mission if they will help them. Please pray that they will not become confused as to what is 'The Truth'. Pray too, that someone may feel called to fill in the gap in this needy place to teach the people about the Lord Jesus. (October 1969)

While the western missionaries played a critical role in opening up and developing West Papua their numbers remained small. In the foreword to *Torches of Joy* Don Richardson places it in perspective.

'It was into this latter field (West Papua) that RMBU placed John and Helen Dekker among the Danis of Kanggime (1960), Stan and Pat Dale among the Yali (1961), Carol and me among the Sawi (1962), Phil and Phyliss Masters among the Kimyal (1964) Costas and Alky Macris among the Lakes Plain people (1967), not to mention dozens of other labourers among these and other tribes.'

All of these pioneers would play a part in Jessie's life, some more than others, and many became life-long friends. Missionaries kept coming: John and Gloria Wilson (1971), Les and Wapke Henson (1977), Orin and Rosa Kidd (1977), Sue Trenier (1978), and Paul and Kathryn Kline who first met Jessie in Karubaga before settling in the Sela Valley for nine years from 1980-89.

By 1972 mission work was expanding on a massive scale as trained Dani evangelists and work gangs moved further and further afield. Jessie's prayer letter of October that year graphically reported the expansion.

We are just 20 minutes flying time from the Lakes Plain area where Frank Clarke and Costa Macris are opening up airstrips to try and reach those who have never heard the Gospel. As they have contact with these new areas, more and more villages are asking for teachers to come in and teach them the Gospel. The need for more workers in this vast new area becomes more and more pronounced.

Almost every week we have sent at least one plane load (about five or six men) of workers down to this area where they stay and work for six months and then return. In the past few weeks Costa has been sending his problem medical cases back to me. Fair exchange I guess! Pray for the safety of the workers in this new area as the Dani folk are working in a very different situation to what they are used to here in the mountains. The Lakes Plain is very flat with many lakes, rivers and swamps. Costa has 500 workers down there organised in building new airstrips and teaching the word of God. One airstrip which is 10 minutes flying will save him 14-days canoe travel.

This was not just the Bible encroaching on Papua on a massive and unprecedented scale. This was modernity crashing in on traditional cultures. Once converted, the Dani embraced their new faith with considerable zest and vigour particularly relishing the chance to celebrate significant milestones in the development of their local churches.

'Hurry, hurry, or we'll be late,' shouted a group of men as they rushed past my house carrying wood, banana leaves and vine. What's the big excitement all about? Today is the Swart Valley Church Conference and they are organising the big feast. All the elders and pastors from Mamit, Kanggime and Karubaga churches come in for a spiritual conference, fellowship and get together. Some 70 churches are involved so that means quite a number of people.

After discussion, a message and sorting out of some church problems everyone gathers together for a feast. The Danis never consider anything is special unless they have a feast to celebrate it. The women folk have been busy all morning preparing it whilst the men sat and talked! (March 1974)

'Quickly bring the potatoes, corn and potato vine leaves' – people running here and there and all intent on the business in hand to get the food in the pits (holes in the ground) with the red hot stones. Men carefully cutting the pig into the right size pieces to fit on top of the piles of vegetables already sitting in leaves amongst the hot rocks. Children carrying

in more fern and banana leaves to cover the top before they are sealed tight and covered again with hot rocks.

What is the special occasion for a feast? - The dedication of the new Karubaga church last weekend. It has been a long-awaited event after working many months hand pit-sawing timber on the mountain sides and carrying it down piece by piece for the framing walls, and selling their pigs and chickens so they would have enough money to buy an aluminium roof for their church.

How many of us would be willing to give a half or quarter of what we possess to put a roof on our church? These folk have done so joyfully and willingly. It is surely a lesson to us to question our priorities on how we spend our money.

Sunday morning saw us all squeezed into the church with about 400 other people for the first service. Looking around one couldn't but be amazed at what these folk had accomplished with just a few basic tools and lots of arduous labour. (March 1976)

Sue Trenier found her friend Jessie completely at home with mission work:

'Jessie was very much called to be a mission nurse. All her nursing, whether it was locals or expats, had a mission to it. She saw it as all part of the whole. In fact she is probably the most holistic person I have ever met. She wouldn't write books about it, but it was a way of life to her and a very effective way because she didn't question, she did, and often reminded me of something my father used to say: 'Christianity is better felt than telt'.'

8. Medical evangelism

They brought in a lady with an arrow in her tummy. She needed a major op. Her bowels were poked in quite a few places. She was amazed to wake up from the op still alive!

She is from a heathen area and this is the first time any of them have come out for medical help. We are praying that whilst she and her relatives are here they might see the difference in our Dani folk since they have trusted the Lord. (June 1975)

While Jessie was a very capable nurse she was also an evangelist, as intent on saving souls as she was on saving lives. Nor was she ignorant of the powerful effect western medicine and exposure to Christian caring could have in the battle for converts. The local animist leaders – witch doctors to Jessie – linked their whole world, including the health and well-being of their communities, to their religious practices and beliefs. When western medicine succeeded where local medicine, customs and beliefs had failed, it undermined the traditional belief system and made people more receptive to Christian teaching.

The flipside of such evangelism was the risk medical failure posed for local clinic workers being trained in basic western medicine when they returned to their villages.

Some will be working amongst villagers where there has been no re-sponse to the Gospel and the people can become very dangerous if someone dies. It is a very big responsibility and they will need much prayer. In the past we have found our medical work has been the spearhead which has opened up people's hearts and doors to the Gospel when they realise that we really care about them. Do pray that the clinic workers will use their position to be a witness to their faith. There are many who are totally com-mitted to their witchcraft and payback system. (June 1980)

Tomorrow will be a very special day for one of my patients as she leaves here after three months of treatment. She was brought in from an area some two-days walk from here, with a badly burnt foot. It was a mess. I had to amputate four toes. The side of her foot was gone and the smell!! Ugh! We have just found out that the day she put her foot in the fire she also burnt her baby alive as a sacrifice to the demon who told her to burn her foot. She felt no pain. Whilst here, she listened to the Gospel and accepted the Lord as her Saviour.

Do pray for Weini as she returns home that she will be able to share her new faith with her family and village who are all non-believers, and very bound up in witchcraft. It has been a thrill to see the change in her over the past weeks. (March 1987)

While Jessie may have initially baulked at being a missionary because she was 'too ordinary' and lacked the necessary gifts, time in the field mel-lowed those views as this extract from her August 1977 prayer letter shows when she shares a quote from Eternity Magazine:

'The nonsense that missionaries are a special people with special strength and unusual devotions has caused enough harm. I've never met a missionary that believes this myth, but there seems to be hardly a church member who does not. Does this mean that people at home are praying for a missionary that doesn't exist? To pray for the strong is only to push a rolling stone, but to pray for the weak is to share in his struggle.'

9. Oubiyo's story

'Selamat pagi,' (Good Morning) chirped a spindly legged little eight-year-old one morning as I approached the hospital. What a transformation had taken place in the face of this youngster who stepped from the plane, obviously terrified, some two weeks previously.

We all have certain incidents, people or events that touch us in a special way and stay with us forever. Oubiyo was one of those people in Jessie's life. His tragic circumstances, healing and Christian conversion encapsulated so much of what Jessie and her missionary colleagues wished to achieve in West Papua.

The story clearly had a great impact on Jessie. It may also have had an impact on many other people around the world. When I casually mentioned at a dinner party that I had started reading and editing Jessie's newsletters it prompted an immediate and vivid account of Oubiyo's story – or at least one remarkably like it - from another dinner guest. While he didn't remember Oubiyo's name, he clearly recalled hearing the story and seeing photographs of Oubiyo's terrible injuries at the South African church he attended as a teenager in 1972.

Jessie's account of her interaction with Oubiyo well demonstrates the causal link between good medical treatment and care and Christian evangelism. There were two versions of this story in Jessie's writings. The reflective version written years later was more complete and better drafted, but it lacked the immediacy of the earlier version banged out on Jess's trusty old typewriter in December 1971.

An orphan from one of the Eastern Highlands stations, Oubiyo had been threatened, kicked and very often gone without food because no one cared for him. He was brought to the missionary in a very sad state with all the fingers of one hand gangrenous and dropping off, and the other hand a weeping mass with all fingers curled up and stuck together. Whatever had happened we wondered.

Then the story unfolded – one of the witches in the village said he had a demon and she was going to burn it out of him. So she forcibly held his little hands over the flames of a fire until she was satisfied. One month later he was brought into the mission station by someone who took pity on him.

'Where do we start?' said Dr Cousens as we looked at the smelling, rotten flesh with pieces of bone protruding through where the flesh had disappeared. After much care and skin grafts he will have some use of the fingers left on the one hand, and with physiotherapy on the wrist of the other, it will become useable again, but all the fingers are gone.

But the biggest joy was watching the transformation in him. The fear and distrust are gone. Pray that the love of Christ may be fully understood by him as he lives amongst us here. There are so many in this land like him, held in bondage by Satan and needing Christ to set them free.

Jess also recounted a sequel to this story.

In the particular area that Oubiyo had come from the witch doctor had repeatedly told the people that if they listened to the missionary's word the pigs would get sick, their potato crops would die and their children would become skinny. This of course discouraged the people from coming to any services that the missionaries held to explain God loved them,

Several months after Oubiyo had been at Karubaga there was a big war at his home village and the witch doctor's wife was impaled with a large spear in her abdomen. The witch doctor knew that he could not help her and asked the missionaries if they could send her to our hospital. This was the first time he had allowed anyone to leave on the plane with his permission. They agreed and called the MAF plane to pick her up and take her to Karubaga. She duly arrived and we operated on her to repair the internal damage done by the spear. She survived the surgery and stayed in one of the hospital huts.

The little boy Oubiyo with his burnt hands looked after her. He was able to explain the routine in the little hospital and how people cared and how he had asked Jesus into his heart and become one of the 'sky father's family'. She could see for herself that the pigs in Karubaga were big and fat. The children were healthy. The sweet potato gardens flourished and she realised that her husband had been telling her lies all those years.

After she recovered from her surgery she and Oubiyo went back to their home village, Naltja. On her return to her people she told them the truth about the way her husband had been deluding them and the fact the people in Karubaga had many fat pigs, many children and lots of sweet potatoes. As a result of these revelations many people began attending the little services that the missionaries held to share the Gospel.

She became one of the first villagers to become a Christian. Some years later the missionary wrote to me to share the fact that the return of the witch doctor's wife to the village changed the attitude of the people and the whole area became open to listen to the Gospel. Many people became Christians and the church began to grow.

10. Death and 'coincidence'

Conclusive evidence that both men have been killed by this cannibal tribe in a small gorge and the bodies carried to a higher grassy slope.

West Papua could be a dangerous and violent place. Missionaries, both the expatriates and their National converts, were threatening local custom and belief and undermining traditional power structures. Inevitably there was a backlash. Most often it was the local converts and their pastors who suffered intimidation and violence from fellow villagers defending the old ways. Few of these attacks, ambushes and murders were widely reported outside West Papua, but it was a different story when expatriates were attacked or killed.

Just days after Jessie's arrival at Karubaga she had been a member of the surgical team that helped save the life of Australian missionary Stan Dale after he was shot five times by Yali bowmen. The event, and Jessie's part in assisting the surgeons, was duly recounted by the wide-eyed and observant young nurse reporting back to her prayer network.

Two years later the tragic sequel to this first attack was played out in the Yali village of Wilboon in the remote Seng Valley, some distance away from the first attack. This time there was no escape for Stan Dale and his colleague Phil Masters who fell in a hail of arrows from tribesmen determined to keep the white men and their new faith out of the valley.

In *Lords of the Earth*, Don Richardson carefully recreated the story of Yali belief and their resistance and later conversion to Christianity, including those fateful days in September 1968 when Stan and Phil made their final trek across the mountains from the missionary station at Korupun, Phil's home station. Stan believed it would be safer to enter the Seng Valley from Korupun, rather than his own station at Ninia.

As they farewelled their wives and families the two missionaries were well aware of the potential danger that confronted them, though confident in their mission. Trouble had been brewing for a long time and was brought to a head when Stan pressured his Christian converts to burn their fetishes, the sacred objects that the Yali believed appeased the spirits and kept their world in balance. Stan was warned that a 'death sentence' had been served on him, but chose to ignore the warning. Now his enemies waited for the missionary's next move to regions that lay beyond their current mission settlements. It was a showdown between two belief systems and the most intransigent supporters on both sides.

The death of Stan and Phil soon made headlines around the world, with Jessie as eager as anyone to transmit the news to her prayer network, registering a series of news flashes in the days that followed the terrible tragedy. It would be almost a decade before Don Richardson uncovered and published the full story of what happened on the trek, but Jessie's prayer letters, drafted from the snippets of news as it came to hand, captures both the urgency, immediacy and horrific nature of the ambush and murder.

26th September

News has just come through from Angurak, a station two-days walk from Ninia, that Phil Masters and Stan Dale had been ambushed on trek yesterday. Two of the carriers fled and brought the news to the missionaries at Angurak. They ran all the way to ask for help. A normally two-day trek was travelled in one day over unused and unknown trails and through enemy territory.

Frank Clarke and Dave Martin were able to speak to the two Dani men on the radio and received their shocked message. MAF was immediately alerted and within minutes a plane was taking Frank Clarke and Jacques Teeuwen into the area. The rest of us at the station gathered together to pray. The Dani folk also gathered together to pray.

Because of bad weather the plane was unable to land, but with the Dani man on board they were able to locate the site where the ambush occurred in very rough country. Frank was able to ask for the aid of a helicopter from TPNG (Territory of Papua New Guinea), and as one was at Tolefomin close to the border it could come next morning to help the search.

27th September

Early next morning the plane again took off and headed for Korupun where the two wives were waiting for their husbands to return from the trek. Pat Dale returned to Ninia to help with the catering for the police and searchers and to be on hand when the helicopter arrived. Phyllis Masters moved to Karubaga to be with her children. We were glad when the helicopter finally arrived this afternoon after some detours because of bad weather. They were unable to begin the search until next day when the weather cleared.

28th September

The helicopter left Ninia early this morning with Frank, Jacques, three police, and a Dani boy on board. A MAF plane circled overhead during the whole proceedings to keep watch on any suspicious movements. This was well worth the precaution as he was able to alert the folk on the ground of warriors approaching from a nearby village.

P.M. Conclusive evidence that both men have been killed by this cannibal tribe in a small gorge and the bodies carried to a higher grassy slope. Their spirits are now forever with the Lord. Please pray for the wives and children of these men, that the Lord will be close to them in these days when many decisions will have to be made.

There was, as Jessie wrote, *the greatest feeling of losses.*

They are planning a memorial service here at Karubaga next week. The night they first heard the news Pat said she could feel the people praying for her and was borne by the prayer. Please pray on. It has been a tremendous shock to everyone. Before she goes Pat wants to finish typing the Gospel of Mark, which Stan had finished translating, and get it printed and in the hands of the people.

There was also anger.

The people of Ninia and Korupun were very shocked of the news and the folk of Korupun were all set to gather arms and wipe the tribe off the face of the earth. Pray for the two little groups of Christians at Ninia and Korupun who will be left without their spiritual fathers.

In the confusion that followed the deaths Jessie made some assumptions that later proved to be incorrect.

The tribe that attacked is not in any way related to Stan's last attack as it was in another valley one-and-a-half days trek from Ninia, and these tribes are enemies to one another.

In fact the Yali, who were responsible for the first attack, had recently sent messages to the Seng Valley tribes urging them to kill any duongs (white people) that came their way. It was a tense, difficult and unsettled time with further violence, intimidation, resentment and fear for Christian and non-Christian alike. Jessie kept supporters updated on the aftermath. Her words cast the event as she saw it. It was a mixture of first-hand knowledge, second hand tales, rumours and gossip.

Still it was exciting stuff for the impressionable young missionary nurse and her equally impressionable team of supporters. You can imagine them being equal parts thrilled and appalled by the bloodlust in the mountains of West Papua.

It was also mistakenly believed, with some reason, that Stan Dale and Phil Masters had been cannibalised by their attackers. Seven years later Don Richardson's investigations, including eyewitness accounts, found that although the bodies had been dismembered and prepared for a feast, there was argument among the villagers on what should happen next. In the end the two missionary's remains were cremated in the normal Yali way to appease their spirits. Meanwhile, more trouble brewed.

Death and 'coincidence'

The people of Korupun began to threaten the Dani workers who were caring for the station and said that if any other white man came into the station they would kill them too. This seemed to be because the death of the two men had not been avenged in their eyes. Hence, a government patrol including Frank Clarke and Don Richardson went into the Seng Valley just one month later.

The Seng Valley people were antagonists and ... twice tried to ambush the patrol on its way into the valley. Peace negotiations failed. The Government had to take strong action and quite a number of people were killed as they attempted to escape from the house into which they had been placed as prisoners. One of the prisoners was finally taken to Wamena which is the closest Government post. The folk around Ninia were overcome with joy at the action that had been taken as this would in some measure protect them. Many who had been too frightened to show any feeling before now expressed a desire to seek the way of Life. (January 1969)

In later, undated writings Jess reflected further on the deaths of the missionaries and its aftermath.

Pat Dale and Phyllis Masters and their children were evacuated from Korupun and went to live on the coast. At the time we wondered what God was doing through this situation but had to remember that God was in control. It seemed all wrong to us but we knew God had a plan to open up this area. When people around the world heard what had happened they were so horrified to think that there were practising cannibals that they began praying for the Yali and Kimyal tribes. Two other mission families were willing to take the place of the Dale and Masters families and work with the people.

Little by little there were signs of change among the Yalis and the Kimyals; they wanted to listen to the message that the men had told them. Different groups from different villages came and asked if a missionary could come to their village to tell them about the great God who loved them. As time went by, more and more of these people trusted Christ and life changed in the Eastern Highlands.

Death and 'coincidence'

There was another interesting sequel to the deaths of the missionaries, a story of redemption and conversion that is also related in some detail in Don Richardson's book. This was Jessie's version as expressed to her prayer supporters at the time.

'Emergency – emergency' MAF Cessna MPH had not had radio contact since 11.05 am. The pilot, Menno Voth, had called to say the weather was bad in the mountain pass and if it didn't clear he would have to turn back. No further word was heard from the plane.

The clouds rapidly became thicker and finally blotted out the entire landscape over the Eastern Highlands as search planes endeavoured to seek the lost plane with the Newman family (Gene and Lois Newman and their children Joyce, Steven and Paul) on board. Early the following morning – in the cloudless sky – the fleet of planes took off to comb the surrounding valleys from which the last radio contact had been made. Each plane carried three or more passengers on board as searchers because the country is steep, rugged and tree covered, and the more eyes alerted the better chance of locating the plane.

Two hours after the search began Paul Pontier called to say they had located the wreckage in the SENG VALLEY – exactly opposite to the village where Stan and Phil had spent their last night on earth.

'Coincidence', you say, Out of hundreds of valleys in those Eastern Highlands for it to be the exact spot of the recent patrol and abounding with hostilities – this is no coincidence.

It seemed impossible that anyone could be alive as the wreckage was scattered down the mountain side and the main body of the plane was burnt out. However, next day a helicopter from Australian New Guinea came over and shuttled MAF personnel (pilot Hank Worthington), *Frank Clarke* (Australian World Team missionary) *and a Ninia Christian Luliap, into the site (Luliap could interpret the local language into the Dani language which Frank could understand).*

A doctor, Jerry Powell, was also on board.

Death and 'coincidence'

The helicopter was able to land quite close to the crash and you can imagine the surprise and delight of the first party who landed to find nine-year-old Paul Newman waiting to greet them.

A few scratches and bruises were the only evidence of Paul's ordeal. Apparently, when the plane finally came to rest, the tail broke off and he climbed through the hole as the plane was beginning to burn. He saw a village close by so he went across the river (a bridge right there across the fast-flowing river). And those same people who had just three months earlier refused the Gospel and killed Stan and Phil, took him into their homes and looked after him. They even got up in the night to put wood on the fire so he wouldn't get cold. The mountains are 6000 feet and over and it is very wet and cold at night.

Paul said that the next day he waved at the search plane but no one saw him as he was away from the crash site on the other side of the river. He cried most of the next morning thinking everyone had left him and he began to wonder if he should start walking to the next station. Then, to his great joy, he heard the helicopter coming and ran to meet it and Hank Worthington who had stepped down from it. A bath – a good bed – food other than sweet potatoes – and friends – did wonders for the lonely boy who spent two nights alone in the Seng Valley.

That wasn't quite how the rescue happened. Paul Newman was in fact some distance away across the valley when the helicopter landed. While Paul, with the help of a Yali tribesman, raced down the steep-sided valley towards the landing site, the helicopter team hastily recovered the bodies of the dead pilot and Paul's parents and siblings and loaded them onto the helicopter. Young Paul was still some distance away as the helicopter prepared to depart the valley. Don Richardson captured the moment in *Lords of the Earth.*

'Wait!' Luliap shouted above the engine's roar. 'Someone wearing clothes is running down that hillside!'

Stunned, the searchers wondered, 'Who on earth could it be?' Hank stepped forward from under the swirling blades to take a clearer look at the small clothed figure racing toward them.

Death and 'coincidence'

'Dear God! It can't be!' Hank shouted. 'But it is! It's Paul Newman!'

At the time, Frank Clarke pieced together details of the plane crash and its aftermath by talking to young Paul and combining his recollections with additional information gleaned from local people through the Ninia interpreter Luliap. Jessie duly reported his findings to those back home.

It seemed that a large cloud settled down on the plane and in attempting to turn and gain height the wing hit the ridge on top of the mountain and they spiralled down to the bottom.

The Seng people told Frank they had looked after the little boy as one of their own. Because of this contact with Paul they now seek to be friends and want a missionary to come in and help them. They desire to build an airstrip and want a teacher to come in and help them read. Coincidence, or the Mighty Hand of God? Only God could change the evil hearts in that place to ones that are now seeking the Way of Salvation. Our God is the God of the impossible.

The seed which has been sown to reach these people has been a costly one. It would seem that God is giving them another chance to hear the Gospel. (January 1969)

Don Richardson's later investigations revealed that it was just one Yali man named Kusaho, not the whole village, who showed compassion for Paul Newman. It was Kusaho who took the boy into his home and looked after him and it was Kusaho who got up during the night and put wood on the fire so that Paul wouldn't get cold. Thus it was Kusaho's actions that provided the bridge towards better understanding between the missionaries and the Yali tribesmen who had originally rejected the new religion and killed the white missionaries.

Jessie maintained contact and friendship with the Dale and Masters families for the remainder of her life, often reporting on their continued involvement in West Papua. Stan's son Wesley following in his father's footsteps, returned to West Papua as a missionary.

I have the Dale family here. Joyce is up visiting where they used to live, and where her father was killed, and then Wesley, wife and baby came along too. I had forgotten what it was like to have a three-month-old baby around the house. (August 1985)

Last month we had Phyllis Masters, her son Curt and daughter Crissie in here for the dedication of a memorial stone for their husband and father who was killed near here some 25 years ago. The people worked hard bringing in gravel the week before so the memorial stone could be built. They worked for nothing because they wanted to share in the special day.

There was lots of reminiscing from the older folk who remember the day when the Masters arrived. After the dedication, the people had a big feast and killed 75 pigs. That is a huge amount for the people here.... In his sermon the pastor said to the people, 'Now we are not to worship this rock. It is here for us to remember what it cost Phil and Phyllis to bring us the Gospel and that God loved us enough to send them here to teach us his love.' (August 1993)

And two years later, this amazing news....

We are praising the Lord for three new visas. One is Paul Newman. He is the boy mentioned in the book 'Lords of the Earth' after he escaped the crashed plane in the Seng Valley some years ago. Now he is coming back with his wife and child to work with RBMU. Pray for them as they start language study in Bandung in two months' time before coming to Irian Jaya.

11. Adjusting to change

Changes are in the air again. Conference has come and gone for another year and with it many changes will be put into effect. The most important one being me of course!!

Jessie's writings give a personal insight into how missions operated in West Papua. While based at Karubaga she often filled in at other remote and difficult locations for colleagues who had fallen ill or taken furloughs after their four-year stints of duty. Similarly, others moved about to cover Jessie's periods of leave or ill-health.

Sue Trenier, a long-time colleague, recalls that it was through this merry-go-round of relief duties that she first met Jessie shortly after arriving in West Papua in 1978.

'I had heard about her skills as a nurse when she worked in Karubaga, especially how she had helped when missionary Stan Dale had been wounded in the Yali area. She was making a move to Taiyeve from Karubaga and needed assistance to pack up her belongings ready for the move. Allocated to the task I got to stay with Jessie, for a short time at least, and strike up a lasting friendship. She was eager to encourage me in my early steps as a missionary and she quickly made me feel wanted, busy and useful, important for a new person eager to do something and please. We packed boxes and sorted endless medicines and food stuffs. My next short encounter was when Jessie was actually in Taiyeve and she was called off to look after a missionary family whose child had been born premature and was in an incubator somewhere. I was on a short break (two months) from my Indonesian language study so it was thought fit to pop me down to Taiyeve for part of that time and take Jessie's place. Talk about being dropped in at the deep end, with a few short practical instructions she was away and there I was trying to fit into Jessie's shoes.'

After Taiyeve, Jessie and Sue ended up living and working in the same area, Sue at Soba in the Eastern Highlands and Jessie a short distance away at her new posting in Korupun – but that was all in the future. First Jessie had to serve her time in Taiyeve, and in May 1978 gave her praying friends an insight into her own movements, and by extension, the operation of the mission service and the difficulties encountered by missionaries going about their work. This excerpt shows the tremendous geographic, ethnic and cultural diversity that missionaries had to adapt to as they moved around West Papua.

Different locations: Yes, I am on the move again! This time just 15 minutes flying to the north (but 10 days walk for the Danis). It would probably take me three weeks. The two nurses from Taiyeve are both due for furlough while Costas Macris had to go home on an emergency medical furlough which has drastically depleted the Lakes Plain staff.

As there is another nurse due to return from furlough to Karubaga, it was thought that I could fill in here at Taiyeve for 12 months till my furlough.

Different climate: As we came over the last mountain range and left the cool mountain air behind us the heat was very noticeable as we sank lower into the Lakes Plain where the weather is very hot. We could see the heat haze shimmering over the tree tops as we came in to land. Hot, humid and sultry most days there is very little to alleviate the heat. It really saps the energy.

Different people: The Taori people are nomadic and are here today and gone tomorrow. They hunt and fish for their food. They search for wild pig in the jungle and are often gone for days or weeks at a time. There is a large river by the station so they also travel far and wide in their dugout canoes.

Different work*: I will be in charge of the clinic with a clinic worker who has trained at Karubaga. There are also a large number of Dani workers and helpers here so I can always get a bilingual to help me.*

There are 18 outposts and airstrips to be supplied with medicines for the teachers and evangelists to give out to local people. The plane calls at least once a month to supply them with medicines and other needs. These supplies are made up ahead of time and given to the pilot who delivers them to the one in charge. If they have any special needs they can call up on the two-way radio and ask for instructions or help.

Yesterday I went along with the plane to an outpost when the teachers there asked for a nurse to come as he had an epidemic on his hands and he did not know what to do. I treated a number of people and gave him instructions as to what to do and left a good supply of the needed medicines.

Different tribes*: At each outpost the people speak a different language so it is important that the Dani evangelists, teachers and clinic workers learn that language to communicate the Gospel. Do pray for these folk who are living in such isolated conditions, often among hostile people, that the Lord will use them as shining lights in a dark place. It is not easy for them to leave their cool mountain homes with plenty of potatoes to come to these hot and humid places amongst strange people with different food.*

Different hazards*: Because of the numerous swamps close by, the place abounds with mosquitoes of all kinds causing two different types of malaria and encephalitis (this causes swelling of the body). TB is also prevalent amongst the tribes' people. Poisonous snakes are quite common and there are crocodiles in some of the nearby rivers so please do pray the Lord's protection in the days ahead.*

Different co-workers*: Annagret and Jurgen Otterbach are in charge of the church work plus numerous other details. Jessie and Marilyn Loffer and Bill and Bonnie Rush are the pilots and their wives are all involved in the Regions Wings flying program. Mavis Honnecher, the bookkeeper, takes care of all the correspondence, finance etc. We also have several*

Indonesian families who take a large share in running the program and caring for the children's hostel.

In her October letter she provided a similar insight into the aerial mission work undertaken by her and her colleagues flying out of Taiyeve, with its 13 different languages at 18 outposts.

I have just returned from a stay at the outposts and am weary, dirty and very hot. Working from one airstrip to another makes for a very exacting but challenging day. The teacher and evangelist had been warned by radio that we were coming, so dozens of people crowded around the plane as we skidded to a halt. All the people with medical problems were there to greet us when they heard that the sisters would be on board.

This one had been burnt badly some weeks ago and it hadn't healed; this one had ulcers in the mouth; this one has a strange rash; this one has a swelling in his leg; this one a swollen arm; and so the voice of the evangelist goes on as he translates from the local language into Dani for me as we see hosts of patients.

Chaos; as they all try to have priority and are pushing and shoving to be seen first and maybe get an injection. Injections are special and a cure for all ills in their estimation. Slowly we straightened up as the last patient is seen and we quickly pack up to be on our way. Everything stored away when yet another patient arrives. Could I please see him as he has a pain in his chest? So we unpack again to see the late comer.

As we race down the airstrip, wave goodbye to all the faces and buzz off into the sky we are reminded again of the vast responsibility the teacher and the evangelist has in that village. They sit and live with the people. They are the only close examples of Christianity that they see and know. They learn the language. They teach and preach the love of Jesus.

The plane is now headed towards another airstrip. Just four more to go today. The hours creep by as we come and go from place to place until about 3 pm when we are finished our schedule and head for home. Soaked to the skin from perspiration after working in the hot sun, feet literally caked with mud from the squelchy airstrips, we are looking forward to a hot shower and a cup of tea.

Adjusting to change

Tomorrow we start again on the radio with the medical problems from the other airstrips that didn't get visited today. To try and decipher what is wrong with them without actually seeing the patient isn't always easy. Then explaining to the teacher what drugs to give and how to use them is something else.

12. A new challenge - Korupun

*Many of you are aware that I will be returning to the Eastern Highlands
and life there will be even more isolated than previously.*

Jessie's first posting at Karubaga lay 71 kilometres to the west of Wamena,
then, as now, the most important administrative centre in the Highlands.
By contrast her next permanent posting of Korupun, lay **88** kilometres to
Wamena's east. The distances don't sound far to the western mind but in
the context of West Papua in the last quarter of the twentieth century these
two villages, just an hour or so apart in the small MAF aircraft, were a
world apart in the context of their place and time. Karubaga was home to
the Dani people who at first reluctantly, then with great enthusiasm, aban-
doned their old ways and became the mountain and valley foot soldiers of
a new and rapidly expanding religion. The Dani converts were at the fore-
front of the evangelical engagement reaching out to near neighbours like
the Yali people, but also to the more foreign environments of the hot and
swampy coastal lowlands. By contrast, Korupun, was home to the Kimyal
people, who were often referred to as pygmy people because of their di-
minutive stature. The Bible came later to the Kimyal than it had to their
Dani counterparts.

Jessie enjoyed sharing mission news of the slow but inevitable advance
of Christianity among the highland peoples with her network back home.

We have been thrilled recently on hearing from Korupun in the Eastern Highlands that a small group of believers have burnt their fetishes. Do pray for this little band of believers because they are often persecuted and ridiculed by the rest of the villagers and much pressure is put on them. It is so much easier to go with the crowd than stand alone against it. (October 1972)

We have been greatly thrilled and encouraged to learn that the first baptism at Korupun will take place this coming week. Some of the Christians in this area have been killed for their faith. It is no light thing they are planning to do. (This is the area where Phil Masters worked before he was killed). (July 1973)

In 1977 when new missionaries Orin and Rosa Kidd arrived in West Papua they were posted to the Korupun station where they became the catalyst for Jessie's own move to Korupun three years later. Rosa recalls the circumstances:

'Korupun had a missionary-trained National clinic worker but no nurse or officially trained medical person. The Dani clinic worker was very limited in what he could do and a lot of medical emergencies would fall on our shoulders. Because of this and the many medical needs in our area, we were constantly requesting the field leadership to allocate a nurse to our station.'

So in 1979, after 13 years among the Dani in Karubaga, and no doubt in response to much prayer and the many requests by the Kidds, Jessie was on the move.

It was at this time that our Doctor at Karubaga had to go home and was unable to return. I was asked by the mission conference if I would be willing to go to Korupun in the area where the men had been killed to open up a clinic for training clinic workers and midwives. If you got sick out there it might be four days walk to a clinic. No roads or ambulances, so you died.

Jessie began a nine-month furlough back in Australia in April 1979 and took up her posting to Korupun early the next year. It is clear from her

January 1980 letters that she was well aware of the isolation, dangers and adversity that confronted her.

My new home is finished and sitting in the middle of a potato patch. I guess I will have to wait until the owner digs his potatoes before I can plant a garden. Hopefully I will be able to grow a few other vegies besides potatoes. The clinic and schoolroom that I need have yet to be built. But I am hoping it will soon be underway so I can get things moving. There has been a lot of unrest in the area and several people have been killed. About 200 people from the Sela Valley have fled to our area for protection as raiding parties from a neighbouring village descended upon them, burnt their houses and threatened their lives if they stayed. One man was caught, staked out and killed. These are our neighbours and need much prayer.

With the cultural differences and limited literacy skills it required patience and perseverance to train the clinic workers.

I began bringing in trainees from the far away villages to work with me for a year and at the end of a year they were expected to know how to diagnose, treat, give the right medications, give injections, fix broken bones, pull teeth and help to deliver babies.

Within a few years there were 30 to 40 clinics dotted around the small mountain villages, staffed by clinic workers whom Jessie had trained. This was the first mass intrusion of modern medicine into the lives of these remote mountain people and the initiative saved countless lives and eased much suffering over the coming decades. In her eulogy Thelma drew from Jess's writing and her own personal experiences to paint a picture of life in Korupun.

'The thing that stands out is her willingness to always be 'on call' to respond without question. The constant cries of 'Yetty,' at her back door (the Kimyal couldn't pronounce the sound for 'J' just like the Danis) or the worried husbands with their wives in labour in the middle of the night, pouring rain. She would pull her tracksuit on over her pyjamas, grab her bag and a torch and step out into the mud. It was no easy task to climb the pole into their small front doors designed to keep intruders out. Jess used to joke it conjured up a picture of the husband pushing her up the pole and through the hole. Once inside there would be the fire… children huddled in the corner and several feet away the pigs. Very difficult in the dark trying to find a vein to put up a saline drip. When we visited it was nothing to find eight or 10 little kids in a circle on her lounge room floor with an inhalation of gum leaves in a bowl in the centre with a sheet over them all. Jess planted and grew the gum tree for the Eucalyptus. She loved her garden.'

Jess's letters from Korupun were as descriptive and colourful as ever.

Just saw some of the elders going off to teach Sunday school so I guess it must be getting near time – now 10.30 am. He was really dressed well – in his skin – and a plastic bag containing his Sunday school book and scriptures under his arm and an axe over his shoulder! Some of the evangelists have just come from the Sela Valley which is the next one to here and said that there was fighting going on there again. Last week one of the Christians was ambushed and killed.... (January 1980)

Where Karubaga was a mission and administrative centre, Korupun was an outpost which Jess shared for many years with the Kidds and her new colleague Elinor Young, an American linguist/translator. Jessie was quick to introduce Elinor to her army of supporters back home. She also painted some wonderful word pictures of her new posting to give them a flavour of the different place and different life she now shared with the Kimyal people.

This week Elinor and I were invited to have 'tea' with one of the local elders and his wife. We duly arrived at 4 pm to share in their big meal of the day. Their little round house is built on a smaller scale than the Dani houses. The roof reaches down almost to the ground so that you have to stoop almost double to get underneath the eaves. The little door was certainly made for pygmy people and not for people my size.

After some manoeuvring I finally got into the house itself. Three quarters of the house was taken up with pig pens and pig honking and squealing were the background music as I began my meal with my back leaning against the sty. This area was about six feet by four feet so we were rather cramped with five adults and two children sitting on the floor to eat our meal. One lady arrived late so she had to climb over the pig rails and sit in with the pigs.

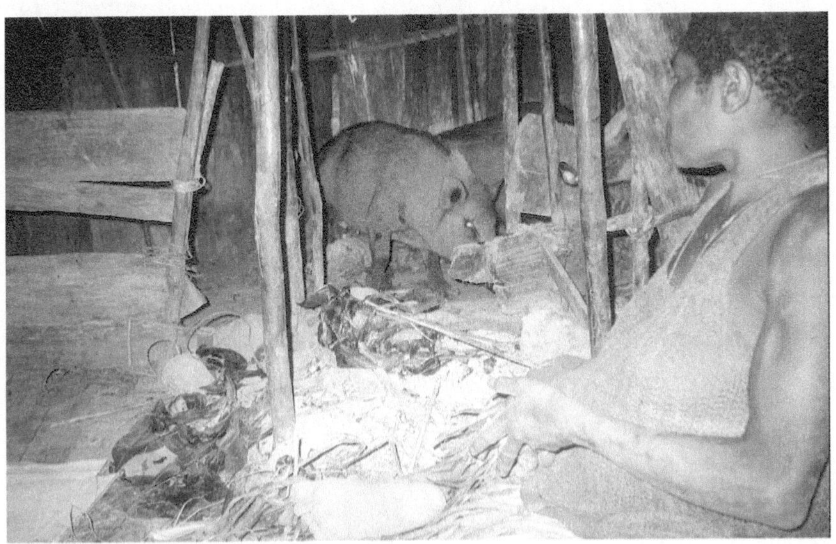

We were treated as honoured guests, and they had cooked sweet potatoes, potato leaves and a few small pieces of pig as a special treat. At night three women and two children sleep in that small area on the bark floor beside the fireplace. No electric blankets there! The women were busy making string from bark after the meal was finished. They had to go almost a day's journey to collect this particular bark, and it makes a very strong string which they use for their pig ropes. I was mostly just a spectator because of my limited vocabulary, so Elinor did all the talking.

Elinor also introduced her to the new routines of life in the high mountains. Learning the new language and local customs wasn't the only steep learning curve facing the new arrival.

Last Sunday Elinor and I went up the closest mountain to church as Elinor wanted to teach one of the elders how to take Sunday school. It sure is a little different from Sunday school at home. Sitting in the sun in the centre of the village with about 30 children grouped around listening intently to the story and watching the pictures. Great competition to see who could be the first six to say the memory verse and gain a picture card as a reward.

Walking on these trails is very different from Karubaga, as the mountains are very steep and the trails just a 'sheep track' of mud and stones. Climbing up through streams, hanging on when there were just toe holes straight up was no joke. Maybe a mountain climber's paradise but!! I finally staggered over the rim to the plateau at the top to see the most magnificent view of layer upon layer of mountains away in the distance. Well worth the effort to get there.

Sunday school over, we headed down, down, down. I sat on my bottom and slid along in some places where it was too steep for me to get a good footing. Crossing the so called bridge at the bottom was an experience – a few round poles lashed together after a fashion, and I was glad to get to the other side of the roaring river.

At the moment I am living with Elinor Young as my house is not yet finished enough to move in. It has a lovely view down the valley of a 10,000 foot mountain with higher ones behind it. They often have cloud and fog clouding their tops and therefore we have very high rainfall.

My house is made of hewn timber from local trees on the outside and pit sawn timber on the floor. The inside walls are of bark. Hopefully the ceilings will be plywood, if and when it gets here, to help with my allergy problems. The front windows are glass louvres and there is plenty of plastic in the bedroom windows. There is a bush septic toilet to go in when we get hooked up to the spring which they tell me is not far up the mountain. The water supply for the kitchen will be from drums which catch rain from the roof; the shower, a bucket.

A wood stove has been bought to go in the kitchen when we can locate some zinc to go on the walls to protect them from sparks. Work progresses very slowly up here so do pray that we will be able to get somebody to help us get all the necessary things done so that I can move in. Then you can consider yourself invited to come and visit me and share in the work here. I would love to have you and visitor's visas are fairly easy to obtain. At the moment I am supervising the clinic here and three out-clinics in the other valleys. There is still a lot of unrest in the Sela Valley and there has been continued fighting on and off since I returned. (February 1980)

Orin and Rosa Kidd were excited to have Jessie join them and welcomed her contribution to the mission team and the Kimyal community.

'We were thrilled beyond words when the Field allocated her to minister with us in Korupun. One of the marks of a good missionary is the ability to adjust. Making a move from one tribal work and language to another is no small undertaking, yet Jessie took up the challenge with her whole heart. She started Kimyal language study and initially used Elinor, Orin or myself to help her with the translation. She was also able to use some Dani and some Indonesian to communicate.'

Jessie's may have been a simple house but it took a long time to complete. It wasn't until October 1980 that she informed friends and family she was in her own home again.

At last the long awaited day has arrived, and I have moved into my own house. It is still far from finished, but I do praise the Lord that at long last it is liveable and I can unpack my own things instead of living out of suitcases and having to constantly borrow from others. I still don't have any water in the house so we are bucketing that. The toilet is set in and I flush it with a bucket. We finally got the new stove in but the chimney is rather short. It barely comes through the roof.

And there were constant reminders that this was a different world.

Elinor and I had the company of two dead pigs as the other passengers on the flight out. One of the Korupun churches wants to buy aluminium for their church roof and asked if we would bring out these pigs and sell them in Sentani for them to buy the roofing while we are here. (August 1981)

After spending three weeks away in Mulia to serve as midwife to a missionary family expecting their second child, Jessie returned to Korupun for Easter.

I was greeted with open arms by the clinic workers on my return, because they had almost run out of medicine. They were all waiting with their empty pill cans to be refilled. They told me there had been a second outbreak of whooping cough in another valley with some more deaths. Unfortunately, not all the mothers will bring their babies in for DPT injections and now it is too late. As I sat in the midst of a throng of dark skinned folk on Easter Sunday morning and listened to their Pastor explaining the wonder of what Easter really means I was thrilled to be part of the Church of Christ in this land. (April 1982)

Greetings once again from wet and windy Korupun. Our dry season seems to have got lost somewhere, so we are enjoying an excess of cold weather. With the continuation of the cold weather we have had a flu epidemic for the past three months which has laid low the whole population for varying lengths of time.... A tablespoon of pure lemon juice and an aspirin is great medicine. (November 1984)

The missionaries had to weigh all passengers and luggage that were to travel on the next day's plane. Sometimes the manifest included pigs, dead or alive to be placed in the pod under the plane. Jessie wrote: *when they realise a plane is due they rush up with all sorts of gifts for their friends in Wamena. It is very hard to convince them they have to stay under the limit.* (1986)

Government services began to follow into areas pacified by the missionaries. Korupun was no exception. By July 1989 a government primary school supplemented the literacy and other education services originally provided by the mission.

Last week we attended the first graduation ceremony of the grade six students of the Indonesian primary school here. It was followed by the pig feast. Thirty students sat the exam and 21 passed, so there was great excitement. Most of the students have now begun the long seven-day walk to Wamena to get enrolled in the high school there. (July 1989)

On 14 May 1991 Jessie completed 25 years as a medical missionary. Her colleague Elinor was nearing the end of her time in West Papua. Small in stature, the result of polio as a child, Elinor could not walk very far and by this time travelled around perched on a makeshift arrangement of hessian supported by long poles on each side. One man on each corner carried this on their shoulders. Thelma recalls that they would often run flat out: 'This appeared very precarious but she loved it!' Unfortunately Elinor's health was deteriorating irrevocably.

Elinor went home in August to get some help for the problem she has been having with severe pains in her knees. After many doctor's appointments, X-rays etc. the results are not good. She has post-polio syndrome which has also affected her lungs, arms, possibly her heart and her knees. She is also using a special wheelchair. It seems very uncertain that she will ever be able to return to Irian Jaya. Do pray for her and for the unfinished Kimyal translation. (October 1991)

Around this time the Kidds were among a group of missionaries who had their visas withdrawn and Elinor's departure meant Jessie would be the only expatriate in Korupun for lengthy periods of time. She knew how difficult this would be when she returned from furlough in late 1992.

Please continue to pray for me as I get settled in again and also that I will not get too lonely by myself.

As always, Jessie kept her network well informed of life, colour and progress in Korupun.

Several weeks after I returned from Australia, Korupun was once again the venue of a large church gathering. This time the Kimyal area churches were officially welcomed into the larger Irian Jaya Evangelical Church body. About 2500 visitors arrived, including government officials from Wamena and delegates from other tribes. A feast followed and many of the people were dressed up in traditional dress – or lack of it – for the occasion. Beautiful head dresses were made from the yellow bird of paradise feathers. They danced and sang until they were hoarse and legs tired. We needed ear plugs. (January 1995)

Excitement is in the air as Indonesia celebrates 50 years of Independence. Flags of all colours are fluttering along all the streets (even in Wamena). All the homes and cars have a red and white Indonesian flag flying. All kinds of special activities are planned for the week of 17 August. Korupun of course is far removed from all these festivities and so life goes on as usual. (August 1995)

13. Through others' eyes

'Yetty nekna' – Jessie is sick. Unfortunately Jessie has contracted hepatitis A and asked the four of us to put down our impressions as visitors.

In February 1989 Jessie's sister and brother-in-law Thelma and Jim Minto and friends Laurel and Jim Thiessen visited Korupun. At Jessie's request they provided an outside perspective of missionary work in the remote mountains and their insights were shared with Jessie's prayer network.

It is February, the so-called 'dry season'. Firstly Korupun is situated in the floor of a valley surrounded by steep cliffs and tall mountains which are more often than not shrouded in clouds and mist. There is scarcely a flat piece of ground anywhere, it is all up and down. There are 38 water-falls around the perimeter of the valley, some small, others falling many hundreds of feet, absolutely spectacular. A continuous background sound of raging rivers is present and it rains every day, over 800 millimetres a year. This combination of mountain and rain creates mud. In fact mud is a constant companion and good boots are essential.

The people are delightful with an engaging sense of humour, and no one passes without greeting. They work very hard on their sweet potato mounds and their prized shovels gleam like stainless steel from use. When the people who have virtually nothing share with you what they have it is a very moving experience. Jim and I helped out with numerous odd jobs and the frustration of such isolation becomes apparent. There is no convenient hardware store nearby! Elinor waited four years to have her kitchen bench re-laminated. Jessie has to continually go outside to turn off the pipe which feeds into a drum, which in turn feeds her toilet system. We were able to fit a new stopcock for her and tidy up Elinor's kitchen and bathroom amongst other things, but could have spent more time doing more of the same. Someone remarked to us: 'The missionaries have to be disciplined or they can spend 100 per cent of their time just living and get no work done.' It is one thing reading about their work and quite another to experience it first hand and we have unbounded admiration for those people and the work they are doing.

Living in Korupun is on two levels, neither modern. On the higher level it is basic nineteenth century accommodation for Jessie and Elinor. Pit sawn floor boards with gaps between, palm internal walls which offer little privacy, wood stoves and bucket showers. The only modern concessions are a flush toilet, fed from a recently installed hydroelectric plant, and corrugated aluminium roofing.

The lower level is almost prehistoric; the local accommodation is circular huts and hand-hewn timber with thatched roofs. Aluminium roofs are highly prized (and priced) as it allows a church building to be large enough to accommodate the village attendance or the clinic to collect fresh water. The local people carry their possessions in a net bag hung off their heads, their water is from the many surrounding streams, their food mainly sweet potato, the occasional pig or chicken and a variety of indigenous plants. Their warmth, light and cooking is provided by an open fire.

These three weeks have been a great adventure, an incredible holiday. The first thing you feel is the love of the Kimyal people for Jessie and Elinor Young. We went on a trek to two nearby villages, about four hours of steep climbing and descending cliffs and negotiating scary bridges. These villagers so anticipated our visit (Jessie, Elinor and us four) they repaired the bridges, built ladders on the steep, steep parts, and prepared a feast at both villages. They vacated houses for us (except for the fleas) and had special toilets built for our use. When you realise how few possessions these people have, it really was 'the widow's mite'. I spent a lot of time with a lump in my throat.

There were many touching moments. On the way over we were half way up the mountain and exhausted, when the local pastor suggested we should pray. So there on the side of the mountain he thanked God for the people who loved them enough to come to their village and for the strength to get to the top of the mountain. With Jessie we ate the local vegies, mainly pork for meat (pork spaghetti, pork rissoles, pork pickled, stewed etc.). The house girl gave us a chicken which we had to cook for four hours!

By comparison in Australia we have so much, and yet we are so quick to complain. I wonder what Jessie thinks when she comes home. She doesn't waste a single thing. When Jessie became sick and went over to Sue Tre-nier's at Soba, Thelma and I were left to run the house for a short time. We decided to cook a meal and invite Elinor over. First we thought we would fix a banana cake which took us nearly all afternoon to organise. What nearly put us under as we were ready to put the cake in the oven was to discover that the fire had gone out. After 30 minutes (Thelma blew and I prayed) we got it all under control. A fairly simple meal was a marathon effort under these conditions.

A lasting memory was coming in and going out of Korupun airstrip. It had two bumps and gathering speed for departure take-off was akin to a roller coaster with a gorge and cliff directly in front of you, then that quick right hand turn with no room for error. We all developed white knuckle syndrome. Those pilots are a race apart. There were many stories told of cool heads and remarkable skills in terrifying circumstances. We were very grateful for the good weather and safe travel. On one occasion the he-licopter we had been travelling in broke down and the pilot found metal fatigue in the tail rotor.

This country has been described as 'the end of the earth and an hour beyond'. Living with the remoteness and the inaccessibility we were amazed at the resourcefulness, patience and flexibility of the missionaries, isolated, but with little privacy, constant demands on their time, always faces at the windows, bodies at the door, someone constantly at your elbow, all requir-ing patient help and care.

Jessie and Elinor speak Indonesian and the local Kimyal dialect. They have done a great job in maintaining the people's culture, self-sufficiency, and self-esteem.

In late 1992 it was another sister Vera and her husband Ken who visited. Their reflections give us further insight into Jessie's world.

To see photos and coloured slides of the areas where Jessie has worked is one thing. To experience it and to breathe in its atmosphere has lifted our understanding far beyond what we had imagined.

To have your hand taken by a small boy in the Wamena market. We could not communicate verbally – his eyes said it all. He saw how much more we had and knew how little he had. Yet to respond to individuals was difficult without being swamped by dozens more in similar circumstances.

To fly through thick clouds along lengthy valleys, flanked by mountain peaks rising above 10,000 feet. Then to fly above these clouds, seeing only the mountain tops, before descending through the clouds again to make a landing. Such was our experience when flying from Korupun to Soba in a MAF Cessna. How we appreciated the skills of these pilots.

To talk to three missionaries about their experiences when their mission stations were hit by earthquakes – Art and Carol Clark at Lolat in 1981 and Sue Trenier at Soba in 1989. We saw much evidence of how mountains were carved up and stripped of all vegetation. We were told of tragedies as well as remarkable rescue operations. We sensed the traumas these missionar-ies experienced as well as the tower of strength they were to the people as they tried to come to terms with all that destruction and its traumatic aftershocks.

Living with a missionary can mean – seeing her drool over a cherry ripe – seeing your gift of rice bubbles for breakfast bought at a local su-permarket at a price missionaries cannot afford, turn out to be stale. Hear the concerns of missionaries after deadly snakes have been killed in the yard where their young children play. Hearing a missionary double check a weather report that it's OK to fly to her area when all other areas are closed. Seeing a missionary being polite when a tourist criticises her for 'spoiling the area' with European buildings, then ask where the shop is to buy water bottles. (Late 1992 - early 1993)

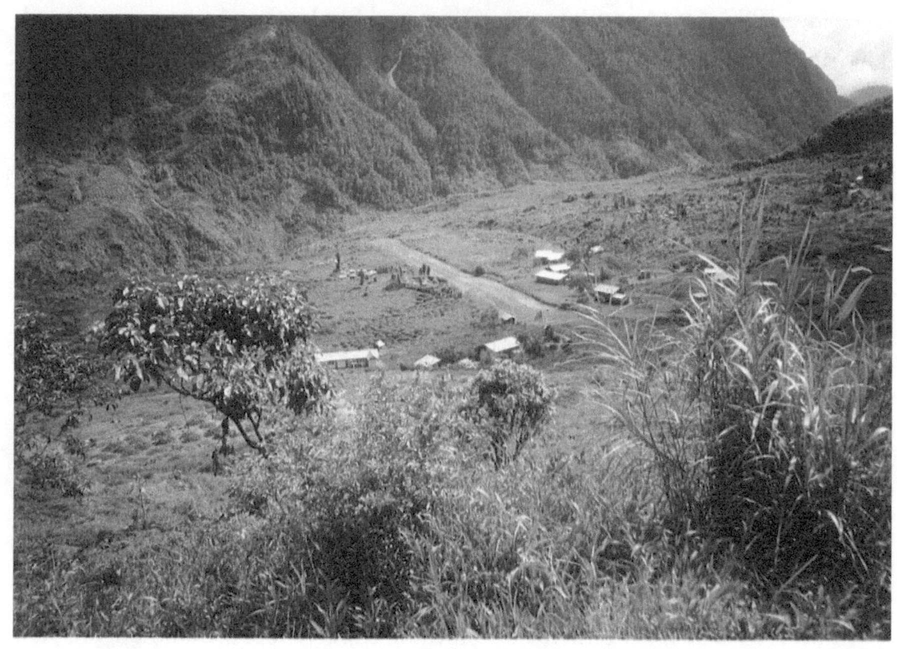

14. Clinic workers

'Jessie worked a medical revolution among the Kimyal people.'
– Sue Trenier

The missionaries were often the first contact tribes' people had with the outside world. Government services were almost non-existent when the missionaries arrived, and there were no modern medicines or medical services. So the missions developed a very practical and innovative model of health care, training some of the best and brightest young men to work as paramedics in their remote home villages.

People often asked me why I didn't train girls. When we suggested it to the local pastors they said, 'No. The girls are too dumb and stupid to learn. Train the men.' Of course they wanted the job and prestige of being a clinic worker. I knew that if I pushed for women trainees they would not be accepted.

The care provided by clinic workers was very basic but effective. In both Karubaga, and later in Korupun it fell to Jessie to do most of the training. Rosa Kidd recalls:

'One of the first things Jessie did was start a training program for our local people. This meant that we would have trained Kimyal clinic workers for a good number of the villages. Most of them did not have a clinic worker at all so this was greatly appreciated. Among other things, Jessie also gave us, her fellow team members, training on how to suture, give shots, do skin grafts, apply a proper bandage, deliver a baby, and diagnose and treat diseases common to our area. She was our constant source for medical knowledge.'

Training clinic workers was a practical, if less than perfect, solution to meet a great need. It required infinite patience and great commitment, for while the candidates for training were usually well chosen, intelligent and capable young men, the concepts underlying western medicine were completely foreign to them. The training process remained remarkably consistent throughout Jessie's service, with Jessie reporting the same difficulties with her early classes in Karubaga, as with her final classes at Korupun almost 35 years later.

The slip-ups, frustrations, cultural misunderstandings and comic moments became part of the banter in Jessie's letters with each new intake of trainees unleashing a fresh round of mix-ups. The ever patient Jess took it in her stride, making light of her difficulties and sharing some humourous moments with her network of supporters.

'Yetty, my temperature is 102 degrees,' said one of my clinic workers one morning in class. Each Monday I teach all our eight clinic workers from the outposts. At the moment they are struggling to read a thermometer. Held upside down, sideways, and back to front it is no wonder some of them came up with the weirdest readings. On the whole they are a bright lot of men and learn quickly. With no text in Dani they have no real reference books so what they learn and write down in class is their library. (June 1972)

'Yetty his blood pressure is 170/100.' As the normal Dani blood pressure is around 100/60 this was rather startling news. 'Take it again just to be sure,' was the answer. He did so and with an embarrassed grin said it was now 110/70. Emergency – no – just teaching the clinic workers to use a sphygmomanometer with rather amazing results. (November 1975)

Most of Jess's trainees had little formal schooling. They came from villages with no running water or electricity. They had no grasp of concepts underpinning western medical thought, yet they were driven by a deep sense of the good they could do with their training as well as the responsibility that went with it – as was Jessie.

'Now what do you do if a man broke his leg and you are far away from the clinic?' 'What do you do if a man falls out of a tree and hits his head on a stone and lies like one dead?' 'Whatever are you doing?' Striving to clarify in the clinic workers' minds what needs attention and what they can safely cope with on their own. Do pray for me that I might be able to make these lessons clear and simple, yet deep enough for them to grasp easily.

Each week the men came in from their outposts with stories of people they have seen and treated. Often they bring in a patient that they have been puzzled about for me to check and explain what to do. Next time they will know what to do themselves. One of our clinic outposts is eight hours walk away and it is a long way to carry someone on a stretcher. The people still relate all their sicknesses back to some old arrow wound or injury and one has to sort out the real needs from the past history. Sometimes this is hard for the clinic workers who have been brought up with this same kind of belief and it is hard to shake. (November 1975)

How do you explain to someone what is oxygen? You can't see it, smell it or feel it. They don't even have a word in their language to describe it. This is just one of the many problems that I have run into in my clinic workers' training class. Starting from the grassroots level has its problems. 'Why shouldn't I wipe my nose on the back of my hand?' 'Why shouldn't I pick up pills with my toes, they are just as good as my fingers!' Please pray that I will be able to make things clear and simple for them that they will understand clearly and remember what they have learnt.

In many ways they will have more responsibilities than a nurse back home. What do they do if you break an arm or leg? What do they do if a woman has a baby and the afterbirth doesn't come out? Call the nearest doctor? They may have a five or seven days walk to me let alone a doctor. These and many other things they have to grasp and remember. People's lives may depend on their ability to cope in an adverse situation.

In some places where they will be going it may even endanger their lives if someone dies whom they have been treating. Would you care for that thought at the back of your mind as you did your best to help someone? So often they come too late to be able to help them and often they have tried their witchcraft first and when that fails they come and try our medicine. (October 1980)

The other day they left the tap on in the clinic and wondered why there was no water in the barrel the next day to wash their hands. We catch water off the roof in drums. Then surely, if someone is very ill, you would of course give them a double dose of medicine to make them get well so much more quickly. It's no wonder that my hair is turning grey. (May 1981)

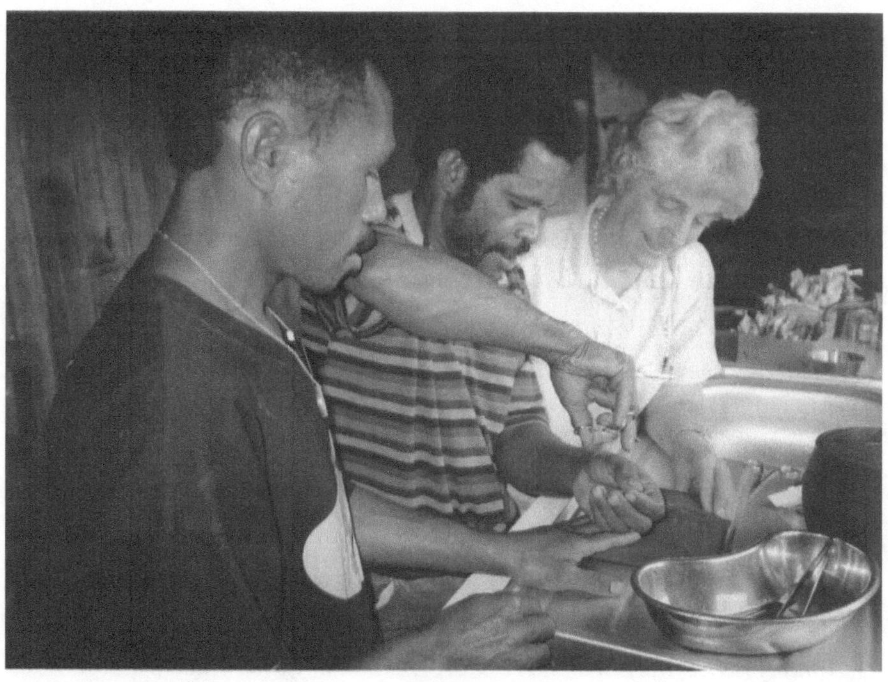

But if the training of each new cohort of clinic workers produced similar difficulties and frustrations, it also produced similar, positive results that greatly improved health care in the highlands and provided a network of trained and willing people to treat injuries, diagnose ailments and undertake vaccination programs when deadly epidemics threatened.

<h1 style="text-align:center">Clinic workers</h1>

A couple of weeks ago we found that the whooping cough had hit a village a day's walk from Korupun and six babies had died. I felt sorry for the clinic worker as he did not know what to do. We were all gone and nothing he did helped. I quickly sent medicine across the trail and there have been no further deaths. (March 1982)

I have begun to teach my trainee clinic workers how to suture up wounds. They have been diligently practicing on lemons to get the right technique in tying knots with a needle holder. At the moment they are still all thumbs, but trust they will improve. People have a little more feeling than lemons. (April 1982)

Jess also realised that in the clinic workers she was leaving a permanent legacy of care that would outlast her time in the mountains. The government also recognised the quality of their training and the value of the health care they provided.

...after much hassle and paperwork, two of the men whom I have trained have finally been accepted by the government as village health workers. This means they will receive a small wage each month. It also means that if we have to leave the country they will be responsible for the medical care here. Do pray for the clinic workers as they have a big responsibility. (March 1985)

The government has decided that the clinic workers, who have had their application in for some time to be registered, are to receive a wage from the government. They have to be in Wamena in two-day's time. Panic. There was no way they could walk from here in two days so we tried to get a plane for them. We just hope it works out. They will be most disappointed if they can't go. (June 1985)

We just got word that two more of our clinic workers are to receive a government wage. They went off to Wamena this past Saturday. It will be a big experience for them as they have never been away from Korupun to a larger community. They have never seen a car or truck. It will be amazing for them. I hope they don't get their money stolen. (1986)

At the moment I am endeavouring to teach two men from Sumo in the lowlands to be clinic workers. (These two men from the Momina people were the first Momina trained as medical workers). *They, of course, do not know or understand the local language so I had to get out my rusty Indonesian and polish it up. It has been very hard for them as they are used to a hot climate and Korupun is just the opposite.* (March 1986)

I now have three men that I am training, so would ask you to pray for them as they grasp all these new names of medicines and when and why they should be given. Why it is important to give fluids to people with diarrhoea etc. One of the outpost workers came in and said he had a child come who had been hit in the head with a piece of wood. It had split his scalp open. Because he hadn't come in for treatment the flies got in and it was crawling with maggots!! What should he do? One never knows what will happen next, and it is hard to give them a comprehensive training in all the things that might happen. (March 1987)

Money was always tight and there was little government help, so the clinics had to be supported by the local community. The men trained with Jessie for a year. Their local village or community had to agree to support them and raise the money for a simple building with an examination table, shelves and bench tops. They were also required to have a metal roof to collect clean water. The village often paid by instalments. They would meet the plane as various pieces and components were flown in and carry them on their heads to their village up to eight days walk away. They truly valued their local health service, primitive and basic as it was.

Next week we are opening a clinic across the Dagi Valley. They are putting on a big feast. They wanted to know if we couldn't get the helicopter would I walk over. It would probably take me 12 hours. I think my old bones wouldn't walk that far now so have to hope the helicopter is around this area. (March 1987)

The church has chosen three new trainees to start next week. Pray that I might have a good rapport with them and that I will have the patience to teach them over and over the same things. (January 1989)

But there were also many moments of triumph when clinic workers successfully put their training into practice.

For part of the time when I was away Elinor had the Johnson's triplets stay with her. The day after I left Korupun they were all practicing doing their cartwheels on the lawn outside Elinor's house, when Karen fell and broke her leg. After one horrified look at their sister the girls rushed inside to inform Elinor who thought they were pulling her leg! Within minutes the head clinic worker, Sabil, and one of the pastors were busily reducing the fracture and putting on a splint. It was too late in the day to call for a plane so they had to wait till the next morning. She was taken to one of the mission hospitals for an X-ray. They found that Sabil had done such a good job that it didn't have to be touched, and they just put on a plaster. When they told Sabil that he had done such a good job he wore a big grin for the rest of the day. (September 1990)

A lab technician recently came to Korupun for two weeks to give a crash course (to Amop and Abogen, two of the clinic workers) on how to use a microscope. They are doing well. I did wonder how the people would react when they were asked to bring specimens. After the initial shock at such a strange idea it worked well. The other day nine little six-year-olds appeared at the clinic door amidst much giggling they all held up their little offering tied up in a green leaf. We have found that two thirds of the population have amoeba. We were also horrified to find that all the drinking places are contaminated. (October 1991)

Drugs and equipment were always in short supply, so Jessie was nothing if not resourceful, bringing a touch of Australia to the mountains to ensure supplies of eucalyptus were always on hand.

The people in Sela are very anxious to dig out the airstrip from under the mud. But they needed some direction to make it straight. Last week Mike Akenbach and I went over in the helicopter for him to stake out the strip whilst I went around to visit some of the new clinics that have been built. It was good to see the workers in their own situations. I gave each of them a gum tree to plant near the clinic and later on they can use the leaves for inhalation. I wasn't able to visit them all as the weather deteriorated and we had to quickly come home. (October 1991)

Kabeyabe who is one of the clinic workers came with great apologies. He told me that two weeks previously he had been called to a village to treat someone who was ill. He had to cross a river. There had been heavy rain the night before and the river was swollen. He tried to cross it but got swept away in the torrent. He cried out to the Lord to help him. He then started to drift towards the branch of a tree that was overhanging the river. He was able to grasp it and eventually dragged himself out. He lost his net bag with all his precious possessions, needles and syringes in it, but was still alive. (March 1994)

Pray for the 10 new clinic trainees whom I have started to teach. They are from a wide area and some have a slightly different dialect. They all understand each other, but I often have to get them to explain different terms they use which are unfamiliar to me. They are all keen to learn. Some have had to be taught how to open a door which has a door knob, turn on a tap AND turn it off again. Everything is new and strange to them including the concepts I am trying to teach them and why they are so important. Their eyes nearly stood out like stalks when I explained about the habits of flies and the life cycle of the round worms in relation to their hygiene. We have lots of laughs. So many different personalities it is interesting to see their reactions. (March 2000)

I arrived back in Korupun to a great welcome as if I had been gone a year instead of three months. The clinic trainees had all walked back from their villages and were ready to settle down and study. I think they were made aware of the things they didn't know when they had the responsibility in their own village. This week they have been trying to take blood pressures. I am glad my life doesn't depend on their results at the moment. Then we go into suturing and giving injections, a big challenge for them to absorb and practice. (September 2000)

Jessie's efforts paid enormous dividends in health and wellbeing in the villages. Sue Trenier, who shared and witnessed so much of Jessie's nursing ministry, has reflected on the lasting value of her training:

'To accompany Jessie down to the clinic where she taught many local Kimyals to become village medical workers and village midwives was a treat. Her teaching and training was totally practical and many times I saw her make huge pitchers of Oxo soup (from packages her supporters sent on an amazingly regular basis) and had the workers take those pitchers to each village to give to those with diarrhoea. The medical workers to this day in that area know how to treat, cure and prevent severe hydration and are often teachers to the formally trained government medical workers who come to work in the area now who think every person with diarrhoea needs dehydration intravenously, which of course is often not appropriate or possible in the village setting. In more recent years since Jess has left Papua, when I have visited the Sela Valley or Korupun, the medical workers will always have their new stories about how, when they have met a difficult case and didn't know what to do - maybe delivering a baby not going well, maybe a broken bone or whatever - and they tell that they have prayed, suddenly something comes back to their memories of what Jessie taught them to do in that particular case. They have tried it and things have worked out and a life saved!!'

15. Village midwives

When I first went to Korupun I really wanted to train girls to be midwives and to be part of the clinic.

All the men said 'no, no, no, the women are too stupid and they can't be trained.' The men wanted the jobs and they didn't want the women interfering, so I had to let it go. I knew that if I trained the women they wouldn't be accepted; I had to wait until the men would accept it.

Jessie's patience was often tested by the realities of local customs but rarely was the frustration more testing than the matter of midwifery. In this male dominated culture local women were excluded from such learning and using the very skills that Jessie used on a daily basis to ease pain and suffering. While she saved the lives of many women and their babies, both at birth and in the critical days and weeks following – not all births ended well.

The other night I woke up at 2 am with a start to hear someone banging on the door. When I opened up the door the man said that his wife had just delivered a baby but it wasn't breathing properly. When I got there I discovered that it had been a breach birth and although I gave it mouth to mouth resuscitation and drugs it did not respond. It is very hard to try and cope in these little houses with the flickering light from the fire and a torch held by someone else to give light. If they had called earlier maybe I could have saved it. It was the first time they had called me during the night so it was sad that it did not respond. It is very hard to try and cope in these situations. We prayed together before I left. She was one of the few Christian women in the village so I left feeling very sad for her. (January 1982)

Sometimes I wonder if I have strayed into the pages of Gulliver's Travels when a group of our pygmy people gather around and I am head and shoulders above them. It makes me feel a bit like a giant. It is no wonder that these little women have problems in childbirth. Many of them have lost their first baby and others have died in labour before the missionaries moved into the area. This past month I have had to send out two girls to the government hospital for caesarean operations to save their lives. (March 1985)

At the moment I am tube feeding a little baby who is only three pounds at three months. The mother lives half-an-hour away so it is a problem to encourage her to come. So I am feeding the mother too, to increase her milk supply and also to encourage her to come back. (March 1987)

Infant mortality rates were inordinately high. For example, a 1994-95 study among the Dani put the death rate for children in the first year of life at 250 deaths per 1000 live births. Vaccination programs and other clinical support obviously made a difference, but how much more could be achieved if every remote village had their own trained midwife on hand to intervene the moment problems arose and to provide immediate care and advice to troubled mothers. In Korupun the long awaited breakthrough came unexpectedly and helped Jess overcome the male prejudice against educating and training women to be midwives.

I had suggested on several occasions that I start a midwifery course, but the men were not interested until some events happened that made them realise how important it was to train these women. Three days walk away in Gobogdua the pregnant wife of one of my clinic workers, Kabeyabe, went into labour. The baby's hand was sticking out but the baby was not coming. As the labour progressed he realised that the baby was lying crossways (transverse lie) and he knew it couldn't be born normally. He quickly sent a note with a runner over the trail to ask me for a helicopter to take her to hospital. They ran through the jungle day and night for one-and-a-half days to get me the message. Unfortunately the helicopter needed repairs, and it was not flying. I quickly made up some medication for her and sent off a runner over the trail, similar to the Pony Express, or relay runners. All we could do was pray. It was the wet season and it was impossible to bring her by trail.

When I did not hear any news for two days I was afraid she had died. I asked Sabil, my head clinic worker, if he would walk across to be with Kabeyabe if indeed she had died. He said he could get news more quickly than that, so he went up over the ridge and started the bush telegraph going. They shout a shorthand message across to the next valley, then they pass it on, and so on. Within a few hours the message was relayed to the far villages. Another day passed with no word, but then on the second day Kabeyabe himself arrived. He said that when he got the message he realised he should have let me know what had happened. I tentatively asked how his wife was, and he said she was just fine. I then said, 'I guess the baby died.' He said, 'No, the baby is fine too.' I was amazed as a hand presentation is usually a problem for both mother and baby.

He said, 'When I heard the helicopter couldn't come, I sat down and cried and cried, because I knew she was going to die. Then I thought, I shouldn't be crying: I should be praying as God can help me.' Whilst he was praying he remembered what I had taught him, but he was so scared and thought he couldn't do that, so he started to cry again. Then he realised that God would help him. He prayed again. He turned the baby to a breech and delivered it, a little baby girl. At home his wife would have had a caesarean section, or have it turned under anaesthetic: certainly not in a bush hut with animals around her. He was so excited he threw his arms around me and hugged me. He said, 'God heard my prayer, and helped me, and both my wife and the baby are alive. BUT,' he said, 'I realise now we need midwives to help our women. If she hadn't been my wife I could not have helped her, for in our culture it is forbidden for a man to touch another man's wife. We need women trained to help women. Would you start to train our women?' His wife was one of the first people I trained as a midwife, and the last time she came in she told me she also saved a lady with a hand presentation. She said, 'I knew how to do it as Kabeyabe did it to me, and God helped me too.' The midwives used to come into Korupun every few months to talk over any problems that they might have and renew the medications that they used to treat their patients.

Jessie capitalised on the opportunity to train women as midwives despite the patience it required and the inevitable frustrations involved.

Have finally got my midwifery class going after a few problems. One trainee now has a new baby so that comes to class in a net bag. Three are from far-away places so they are really 'green' and we have to start at the grass roots with them. My lessons vary from arithmetic explaining what is a half and a quarter, to hygiene, reading scales and making out charts. I pray they won't become discouraged and I will have patience and insight. (July 1993)

The four women who have started in my midwifery classes are coming along very slowly. Three are from outposts so everything is very new to them. They will also be running the village health program of weighing babies, checking for problems with the babies, teaching the mothers hygiene as well as being midwives. Two of the girls are smart and two very slow which makes it hard for me to teach them, but they are keen. (August 1993)

Around this time the need to train midwives was receiving some high level backing in Jakarta where President Suharto's wife was reportedly promoting a scheme to install a fully-trained midwife in every village within three years. So Jess and her nursing colleagues - Carol from Lolat, and Sue from Soba - were summoned to a government seminar at the home of the Bupati (like a local mayor) in Wamena, a house Jess described as *a lovely home with a beautiful garden.*

Jessie felt the proposal was totally unrealistic because the lack of basic education meant the local women were ill-equipped for the demands of a formal three-year course. Nevertheless the project went ahead with Sue Trenier asked to supervise. Jessie was often seconded to assist.

I made a quick trip to Soba to meet with the coordinator of the new midwifery school that Sue Trenier is supervising there. I will be doing some practical teaching later in the year. My midwifery students arrived back one by one last week. The last one was a week late (It was a three-day walk). (March 1994)

I should have started my new midwifery classes this week but one of the women didn't come. So I asked why, and they said two girls from the village wanted to come and were fighting about who was to come – so no-one came! There is still a long list of women who want to train so we will substitute someone else easily enough. (June 1994)

The long awaited day arrived when my midwifery students finally graduated. They cooked up a big feast for all of us, and then left to return to their villages. From all reports they are doing well. Do pray the Lord will give them wisdom for each case. The other day I heard that two of the girls were vying over who would help with the delivery. We have had to define some boundaries for them. Clean banana leaves and new grass spread on the floor is the usual delivery bed. (July 1994)

After our weekend in Wamena I went into Soba to help Sue with the teaching of the government sponsored midwifery school. The midwife who was supposed to help her went off and got married and never came back. A Dutch nurse (plus her dog) and myself went in to help with the teaching for a week. (February 1995)

My new pupil midwives are settling in. The government has given us some money to help feed some of the undernourished children. They are now running the 'soup kitchen' non-stop all morning, cooking up corn, soya beans, rice, peanuts, spinach etc. In between times we do some classes. (May 1995)

With so many medical and social emergencies to deal with, the students had ample opportunities to learn from very real and practical experiences.

Yokina was one of my trainee midwives and it is very hard to teach people who don't have any books to help them understand things. One day I had just finished clinic and I was up in my house. Yokina rushed up to my house and banged on the door stating: 'quickly, quickly Yetty. There is a lady who has just given birth. She tried to kill the baby by hitting it on the head with a stone and it is not breathing.' I quickly grabbed my midwifery bag and ran down with Yokina to the area where the lady had given birth amongst the high grasses where she couldn't be seen. But someone had noted where she had gone and had followed her to stop her from throwing the baby away. I quickly unzipped my bag and took out a baby suction device to suck the mucous out of the baby's throat and then did mouth to mouth resuscitation and it finally cried. One of the Christian ladies in the village said that she would take the baby and look after it. This is most unusual as they would not normally give their breast milk to someone else's child but because she was a Christian she wanted to save this baby.

The following week I had the midwives come in for their regular monthly debriefing. Yokina came to me very excited because she had been called in the middle of the night to deliver a baby up the mountain. After a long labour the baby was delivered but was not breathing. 'Because I saw what you did to the other baby the other week I did the same thing to this baby and it started to cry,' she said. In their training I had used a doll to teach them this procedure but obviously it had not sunk in because it wasn't a living baby. (Later reflections)

We had all the clinic workers and midwives in for their bi-monthly conference. I had promised to teach them how to put down a gastric tube. After explaining how to do it, we made them practice on each other. This caused a lot of laughter and tears as they found that it wasn't as easy to swallow a tube as it looked. Some were quite hilarious in their actions and comments. I hope they all learned and understood what it was all about and will be able to do it safely to save lives. Then there was the usual scramble to get all their medicines together, listen to all their problems and hear how the Lord had helped them. (August 1995)

We were thrilled to hear that all the trainee midwives passed their final exams. They are part of the government program to put midwives into all villages. Next week the parents of the two midwives from here, plus myself, will be going to Soba to join in the festivities and graduations. They will then go out from Jayapura for a month for practical work before coming home to start work here. They are both only 19 years old. A big responsibility for them. (September 1996)

Graduation ceremonies were always a big deal, and from the tone of her letters Jess was both bemused by the local enthusiasm for the events and excited by the prospect of attending and seeing her young charges celebrate their achievement.

The midwives in the Dagi Valley had been happily planning and shopping for the big day of their graduation for weeks. Questions and answers daily on the radio. Yes, I have bought the rice and noodles; Yes, we can stay four hours; Yes, I have ordered the helicopter for the right day and on and on. Suddenly a bombshell hit when we heard that both helicopters were down and needing parts not locally available. Our flight would probably be cancelled. What a disappointment. Everyone started to pray for the situation and for the needed parts to be found. I told them to go ahead with their festivities just the same. The night before we were to go the pilot called up on the radio and said that maybe, just maybe he could get the parts together, do a test run and still come and get us. I sat by the radio all morning and at noon he called to say they were on their way. He dropped us off in the village and went to refuel. The weather quickly deteriorated and he couldn't get back so we were stuck there for the night. The graduation went smoothly. We gave out their work packs and a message. We were then given a chicken each as a thank-you gift. I stayed the night with Epsin, one of the midwives. (September 2000)

After retiring from active service in West Papua, Jessie kept up with news from her friends and former colleagues. Little pleased her more than news that the network of midwives and clinic workers she had trained were providing an ongoing legacy of medical care in the highlands.

I do praise the Lord for recent news from Irian that the men and women I trained at Sela Valley and Korupun are continuing to work faithfully in their clinics and serving their people well. Sue Trenier was in the area recently to hand out midwifery kits/bags from the health department to the midwives. She wanted to explain how to use the new equipment. She was encouraged to see that both the midwives and the clinic workers were doing well. Continue to pray for Sabil as he continues to have the responsibility and oversight of the 41 clinic workers. (July 2002)

In 1998 Jessie was inducted as a Member of the Order of Australia (AM): 'For service to international humanitarian assistance in the Central and Eastern Highlands of Irian Jaya for more than 30 years.'

The Order of Australia is the pre-eminent way Australians recognise the achievements and service of their fellow citizens. Nominations for awards in the General Division of the Order of Australia come directly from the community.

The midwife program was one of the important humanitarian initiatives that underpinned Jessie's nomination for this prestigious award, one of the highest honours Australia can bestow upon a citizen.

16. Staying connected — staying well

My mail is very spasmodic and some seems to have been lost.

While the western missionaries lived and worked with National evange-lists and local tribes' people, they also maintained contact with the outside world and their own small network of expatriates within West Papua. It took some getting used to because compared to life in their home countries; life in the mountains was remote, rustic, dangerous and difficult.

In the early days, mail could take months to arrive or not arrive at all. In the wet conditions Jess was requesting thongs, footwear that was rela-tively new and as yet unavailable in West Papua. Most of the parcels went missing. Jessie's sister Jean resorted to filling 44 gallon drums with various foodstuffs and goods that weren't available 'out there'. Sent by boat, they often took more than three months to arrive, sometimes failed to arrive or turned up damaged.

I have heard that my fridge has arrived at the coast but have been told it is badly damaged and may not be any use. At long last parcels sent airmail are beginning to arrive. The first I received had been posted five months previously. (Air freight is very reliable and only takes about three weeks. This goes direct to West Irian and not via Indonesia as all mail does). (April 1967)

While basic foods were hard to come by in the mountains Jessie did receive support from her network back home where sister Vera Ewins helped rally the troops:

'Many people have asked me 'What can I send Jessie'. When she was on furlough I put the question to her. Although she was reluctant to answer here are some of her suggestions. Firstly remember – there are NO SHOPS which means you haven't the choice of varying your diet as goods have to be ordered by the case load! So go around your local supermarket and buy a variety of goods in small quantities, i.e. 105 gram tin of salmon, very small tins of baked beans, spaghetti etc. Remember packets weigh less to post and Jessie has to pay freight from Sentani into her on all articles we post. Don't put soap, talc, perfumes etc. in the same parcel as packed food. Wrap all packet foods separately in glad wrap. Cake mixes, instant puddings, packet soups, sweets, chocolates.' (1984)

You will be pleased to know I received a big box of goodies from you when the plane arrived. Thank you for all the special things. They are much appreciated and well enjoyed. (November 1984)

I received two more parcels from you when the plane last came. It is hard to see the labels but I think it was posted in March (five months before). I was very pleased to receive the books as I do need reading material. The chocolate bars and lollies travelled well. The little tins of salmon and lamb tongues are a treat. We had a packet of the Red Dragon long soup last night for tea and enjoyed the change. (August 1985)

We have recently been having problems with Customs changes. It is illegal to send clothing. I am sorry for those who have faithfully sent clothing for the people; we have appreciated it. Other packages have high duty if it is over five kilos. NCV [presumably No Commercial Value] is not accepted as they say you wouldn't send it if it wasn't worth anything. (January 1995)

Jessie was a prolific letter writer. She wrote about five or six personal letters most evenings during her 35 years in Papua, only occasionally missing these writing sessions because of unforeseen circumstances, and had friends in every Australian state and abroad. This was her wider family. She was never idle and used every spare minute to write, though unreliable mail services meant her letters and responses often went astray.

I wrote over 100 letters the week my permit came through, haven't heard from anyone so guessing they have all gone astray. Sometimes if the planes are down or the weather is very bad we will send mail over the trail by carrier if we know a plane is scheduled elsewhere. In February this year I received a fruit cake posted 12 months ago! It tasted OK. (1986)

Communicating with the outside world was a constant problem. Mail was delayed or simply went missing, sometimes by the bag loads it seems. In September 1986 Vera informed friends and supporters:

'Further to Jessie's remarks regarding letters not getting through we have received very few since May. This prayer letter has come via the Philippines. In an accompanying letter to us Jessie wrote: Thank you for your letter that arrived on the last plane. I was rather flabbergasted to hear that you haven't been getting my mail. I am also assuming that you didn't get my last prayer letter written in June either. (We didn't).'

Because of the lack of pilots and planes at present we have only been getting a plane every two or three weeks. My mail has been very spasmodic and some seems to have been lost. If you haven't heard from me please write again as I probably did not get it. Occasionally the next valley has a plane and then I can send mail over to catch their plane. It is a day's walk. (September 1996)

The situation improved little over the years as shown by this email from Pat and Mike Clark to Vera and Ken in October 1999.

'In the last email I received from her (Jessie) a few days ago she said that she has had no mail since her sister died. So I think that she is feeling a little dejected and lonely.'

Jessie's good humour sometimes masked the anxiety that went with her work. In her letters she often reflected on the responsibility of decision making in life and death situations. Sometimes she asked supporters to pray for the community clinic workers and midwives making decisions with their limited skills and knowledge. Occasionally she revealed her own doubts and concerns, for needs were great, resources limited and judgement calls often had to be made.

Last week a runner came from a village eight hours walk away to say they had a lady who had been in labour for three days and what should they do? I quickly sent off the local stretcher, a rice bag with holes cut in the corners to put poles through, to carry her. Also sent a clinic worker with an injection of pethidine for her. I was very thankful when she delivered a healthy baby boy. It is a hard decision whether to call a helicopter or not, they cost so much and especially on a Sunday when the pilot is off duty. (1968)

Such responsibility always weighed heavily on her, even with the great experience that went with her many years of service.

Last week I had a letter from a village three days walk away to say that a lady was haemorrhaging (like a tap). Could I please get the helicopter? The helicopter was in the area and the pilot tried for two days to get her out. The fog would settle down on the village and he couldn't find it. I am thankful that she has improved, but will probably need surgery later in her pregnancy. Do pray for me in making these decisions. It can be an expensive decision if it is wrong. (September 1996)

Jessie, the health service provider, also had her own bouts of ill-health, enduring many of the same risks and the same primitive conditions that affected her patients.

Three months has now passed since it was discovered that I had hepatitis and bed became my constant companion. The first week when I was a lovely shade of yellow, my Dani friends were very anxious, but when I returned to my normal colour they could not understand why I was not working again. (May 1968)

Rest and recuperation were foreign concepts and didn't come easily to the normally energetic nurse.

It seems that I will have to rest more during the next six months to try and get my liver back into shape. This would have been impossible a few months ago, but now another nurse, Mary Freizen, from the Christian & Missionary Alliance (also recuperating from hepatitis and on light duties) has been able to come and help us here in the hospital for four months. It is not easy to sit and watch others take a heavier load. (June 1969)

Shortly before returning to West Papua from furlough in Australia in 1983 Jessie was rushed in for surgery, reporting the experience in her normal, jovial and optimistic style.

My unexpected and sudden visit to hospital for surgery put a very definite end to my jaunting around in such a carefree manner. It certainly was an experience being on the other side of the sheets for a change. I was thrilled to find that the anaesthetist is a Christian doctor. The specialist was amazed by my rapid recovery but I know it was in answer to prayer. She allowed me home on the sixth day after surgery... something she told me she had never done before.

I still have to return to Indonesia on 19 December because my papers expire. Instead of going direct to Korupun I will go to the language school in Bandung for three months. This will be to upgrade my Indonesian while I recuperate. I will be staying with a Moslem family who live close to the school. I understand that the regular meals on the menu are fish heads and rice; so maybe you had better pray for my digestion (or indigestion). (December 1983)

The 'unexpected' surgery was a hysterectomy. While her sisters can't recall the exact details, they think the procedure was performed so urgently because she was returning to such an isolated place.

'Her doctor in Melbourne did express concern from time to time about her returning where she could not have access to good health care. This was particularly so when she had nephritis and really should have had more frequent checks on her kidneys. Amazingly they did recover to a large degree. On another occasion she caught Hepatitis B from a needle prick. For months she dragged herself down to the clinic in the morning and slept all afternoon. I don't know how she

kept going. She was not sure what her condition was and it was con-
firmed by blood test when next she was home. Again, amazingly, she
did not suffer liver damage.' – Thelma Minto

*Yes, I am home again for further medical tests regarding my kidneys.
This time the verdict is I have nephritis (a kidney disease). The specialist is
happy there is no further deterioration of the kidneys but I do have a high
uric acid level that is giving concern and I will need to continue medication.* (October 1994)

Thelma recalls that quite early on Jessie also contracted Filariasis, a
parasite introduced by mosquitoes. The parasites block the lymph system
if left untreated:

'Before treatment was available it was known as 'elephantitis' as
it caused a swelling of the arms and legs to the point you where it
affected mobility. Unfortunately the cure was almost as bad as the
symptoms and many times over the years she would be feeling terrible, recognise the symptoms and take the tablets that left her feeling
wretched for a week - but of course there was no choice. Jess never
considered not going back.'

On 9 May 1996, Jessie celebrated 30 years of medical missionary work
in West Papua. She had arrived as a young woman prepared to live an
arduous life in remote and difficult circumstances. In many ways the physical conditions had improved somewhat from those early years. Nevertheless, hers was still a rustic existence, and the work remained physically
demanding as shown in her report on a trip to Lolat around that time:

*The helicopter dropped us off, and it was due to come back in three days
but due to needs elsewhere it turned out to be four days. We divided up into
teams of three and each team went in different directions to different villages. We walked out to a village two-and-a-half hours away. The trail was
slippery, muddy and steep. We arrived at 9.30 am and we worked non-stop
until 2.30 pm. We had immunised 63 children against TB, measles, polio
plus triple antigen injection. They had prepared chicken and vegies for us
which we were very ready to eat by then. We left at 3 pm. I was tired so it*

took us three hours to get back, right on dark. The last steep climb from the river was the worst. One of the young men pushed and pulled and helped me over the slippery rocks and hard places. I was so thankful for his help, even when he nearly pulled my arms out of their sockets. The old grey mare ain't what she used to be! (May 1996)

Jessie was amazingly resilient coping with a kerosene refrigerator that sometimes needed spare parts. She would write with details and requests and either wait the three months or more for parcels or if anyone was coming to Papua, ask them to bring the parts with them. Fellow missionaries, neighbours or visitors who were at all practical were roped in to help out with anything not working.

Staying connected was a massive undertaking. Jessie's regular prayer letters were distributed to more than 600 people.

17. Clash of cultures and beliefs

The myth that primitive people have such a relaxed, enviable existence away from all the pressures of modern life takes on a very different view when one gets to know their tensions, drudgery, constant fear of evil spirits and the hopelessness of it all that binds these people.

The missionaries who first ventured into the swamps and mountains of remote parts of the island of New Guinea were driven to reach the 'unreached' and be the first to bring the good news of the Gospels to remote tribes' people. Each new tribe was an entity unto itself. The missionaries were also at the vanguard of a much bigger movement as post-war Christianity struggled to reassert itself after the tragedies and devastation of two world wars, a great depression and the post-war ideological struggle between east and west. Christian faith had been challenged and undermined by these catastrophes and Christian churches were re-examining, refreshing and re-inventing themselves to meet the secular challenges to their faith and legitimacy.

After World War Two a new evangelical zeal swept the protestant world. This was the era of Billy Graham, the great Christian crusades and street ministries seeking out the lost and disenchanted generations who were questioning and leaving their faith. The call to overseas mission was embraced by a similar zeal and enthusiasm. The Catholic Church too was probing its own relationship with the modern world at Vatican II to see how best it should respond to the challenges of modernism. These were the times and the context in which the missionaries of West Papua were operating. It is hard to imagine two worlds and two concepts of spirituality more different than that of the western missionaries and the people they evangelised in West Papua and rarely have evangelising Christians been subject to such intense scrutiny of their interactions with Indigenous people.

People say why don't you leave them as they are, they are happy as they are. But once you live with them you find they are not happy. They lived in constant fear. Fear for the spirits, fear of sickness and fear of getting caught by the enemy, killed and eaten. If you got sick you had to give a pig to the witchdoctor then cover yourself with blood and sing and dance all night to keep the spirits happy. If someone died all the close women relatives had to chop off a knuckle to try and appease the spirits. If twins were born, you had to kill one. Either throw it in the river, bury it alive or bash its brains out. Would you like to live in their shoes?

Jessie was an evangelical missionary nurse, not an anthropologist, but she was a keen observer of local customs and duly reported her observations to her prayer network. Often these observations were tinged with her natural optimism, routinely contrasting the joy that came with new Christian values to the decadence and fears of the old ways and religions.

As Christmas draws closer our people are getting excited and planning a big feast to celebrate the birth of the one they now love. Previously they would have had a feast to appease the 'spirits' and for war victories. Since their lives have been changed so miraculously, their motives and attitudes in life have also changed. Now, a feast means a time of fellowship, of hearing the Words of God explained to them, sharing, praying and singing together. (June 1966)

Have you ever attended five weddings in one day? Yesterday we went down to Karubaga church and with joy witnessed the joining together of five young Christian couples. Can you imagine us, sitting on the ground in the dim light of the big square church building with its grass roof, while they solemnly repeated their vows and the elders, equally solemnly, taking the service and praying for each individual one in turn. Shining black faces with wide smiles made it obvious this was a special day for them.... Quite an experience! These young folk have great potential, and now they are marrying Christian wives. What an example they are to others. (May 1967)

The people of the lowlands are very different in attitude, dress and culture. There are just a few who have turned to the Lord amidst much opposition from their families and villages....these new believers are often persecuted, beaten, threatened, and some turned out of their villages for their beliefs. (August 1967)

How would you like to sleep with a skull as a pillow and wake up in the morning with a row of grinning skulls dangling from the ceiling looking at you? This is the case in many of these South Coast villages where the Lord Jesus is unknown or unwanted. Skulls of war victims or revenge parties are carefully polished up and are used in drawing the evil spirits to worship and to help in time of war for these folk. (August 1967)

Other writers of West Papua at this time comment on an abnormally high suicide rate among women. Jessie was no exception.

Just today a woman committed suicide by jumping in the river after a family disagreement. The hopelessness of their lives is appalling.

We tend to see suicide as a malady of modern life with its strains and stresses, so it comes as something of a surprise to see the frequent references to suicide, particularly among young women and girls, in Jessie's letters. Nor do the suicides appear to be the result of the collapse of traditional society under outside pressures, but rather the strains traditional society itself imposes on girls and young women.

A few days ago a stretcher (rice bag) rushed by my door with 20 people in tow. As they passed by they called out, 'Come quickly to the clinic.' A 14-year-old girl had jumped over a waterfall to try to commit suicide because her father was trying to force her into a marriage she didn't want. After checking her thoroughly, she, amazingly, only had a fractured pelvis and multiple bruising. She was shocked and wet through when she fell into the pool at the base of the waterfall.

Trying to get her warm we had to take off layers of wet grass skirts. I asked for something to wrap around her. Two ladies promptly wrapped one of their many skirts for her. Instant dress. We then wrapped her in a blanket. The elders have been counselling with her and her father. Pray for the elders that they might have wisdom from the Lord and that the father will be willing to listen. (January 1995)

One Saturday evening I heard a loud shouting and calling up and down the mountains. It transpired that a lady had jumped off a cliff after having an argument about a pig. They said, 'Of course she died,' when asked. Two days later they came to tell me she was alive. Could I please come and look at her because she couldn't walk. I trekked around the mountain to her village, and after examination decided she had a fractured pelvis, and not a fractured spine which is what I had feared. We sat and chatted and prayed for her. The people told me that in the past that particular cliff had been well used by many girls who were ill-treated or unhappy, as a suicide jump. Praise the Lord since the Gospel has come, it is now a rare occurrence. (Christmas 1999)

The local practice of infanticide of the second twin also caused her much anguish.

Today, a call on the radio from a station in the Eastern Highlands. A missionary calling the doctor to ask what to do when a mother had had one baby and the other twin hadn't come. Impossible for a plane to get in to get the patient out, so instructions were given to the missionary whilst the doctor 'stood by' on the radio to give further help if necessary. Several hours later a relieved voice came back over the radio to say the baby had been born and all was well. But now what? The people in this area are still very much under the influence of evil spirits and if any twins are born, one must be killed. Shocking, yes, but to those people to whom life means, stealing, lying, killing, fear and cannibalism, what is the life of one small baby? Why do missionaries stay in such a dangerous place with no thanks for their help? They have seen the tremendous change in others who have turned from their evil ways to the love of God. A life which suddenly has meaning and a lack of fear of the future is a great and wonderful thing to see. (Circa 1975-76)

There were still tensions between the teachings of the new religion which many Indigenous people welcomed, and the traditional family ties, rituals, responsibilities and expectations.

To realise what a deep understanding these people have of spiritual truths when such a few short years ago they were killing and being killed, in absolute fear of antagonising the evil spirits and fear of the afterlife in case they upset the spirits. Now, the joy and peace on their faces since they have put their trust in the Lord Jesus is something to see. (Easter 1977)

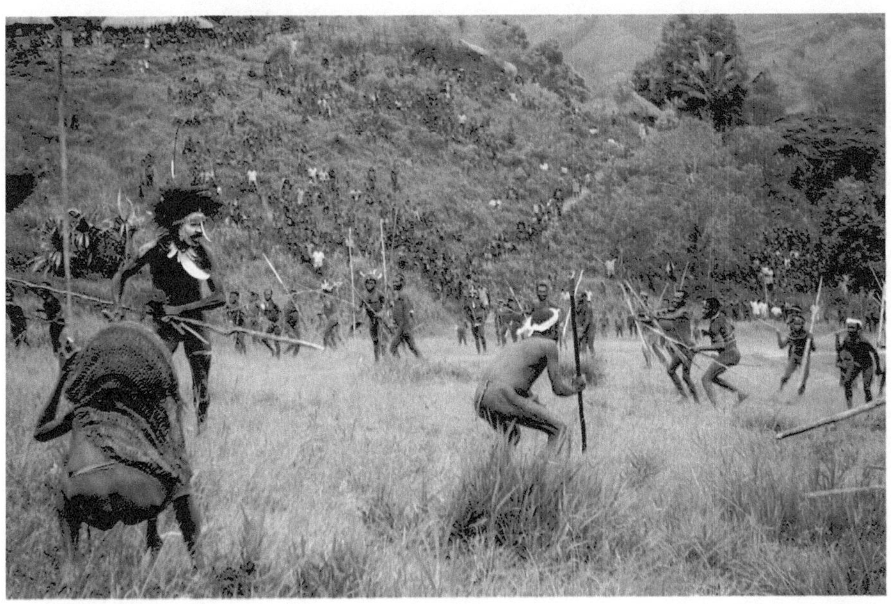

Many of you have been praying about the war that broke out here some months ago involving four villages. Incidentally it caused a lot of extra work for me in patching up the participants. This war was a big disappoint-ment to us because some of our believers were involved and war has been the cause of much heart searching amongst the church people.

Many have come to rededicate their lives, others have come to ask how they can become real Christians and not just as church goers, others to forget old grudges and put them behind them. As God has forgiven their sin, they are now learning to forgive one another. For some this is particu-larly hard for them to do, especially for those whose loved ones had been killed by certain people (whom they know) not to take revenge into their own hands. This is just an infant church and their old ways and witchcraft are very close around them. (October 1980)

Jessie often drew comparisons between the Christian story and the everyday lives of the Kimyal, Dani and other Indigenous people.

The children were huddled together to keep out of the wind, but their eyes were glued to the picture book as the teacher explained the story. So many of the Bible stories they can relate to, as they too have seen people possessed of evil spirits. They have seen them become so strong that no one can hold them back. They know fear, if the spirit's anger is directed at them. (May 1981)

One of the main things that impressed the people about the Christmas story is the humble place of Jesus' birth. They say they can identify with him in this as their women often gave birth beside the pig pens in their homes. They have to clean out their pig pens each day, and they often wonder if Joseph had to clean out the stable before they had a clean place to stay. They say: 'He understands us and the way we live because He too began in a lowly stable just like our little houses.' (January 1982)

As usual in places where Christianity spread its messages, many local traditions were adopted and incorporated into Christian rituals.

A couple of weeks ago we had two weddings in the new church. Their weddings are a little different to ours. They call a wedding 'being prayed over'. All the girl's clan sit together and the boy's family likewise. Usually they sit separately, men on one side and women on the other. At the appropriate time all the bride's clan have to put up their hands to say that they agree with the marriage and the marriage payments have been made. Then similarly the groom's clan put up their hands to say that they are in agreement with the marriage. (August 1991)

The coming of Christianity dramatically altered the social balance of communities. It is interesting reading through Jessie's accounts how often church elders took on the role of conciliation in tribal and family disputes, trying to find a solution that met the needs of traditional lore and retribution for wrongs, but in a Christian context – not an easy task.

That week one of the clinic workers came to tell me that premature twin boys had been born in his village and the mother wanted to keep both. I was thrilled because they usually throw one in the river or bash its head in. One baby was one kilo and the other one and a quarter kilos. Each day they would bring them down the mountain for me to tube feed them. I was encouraged when after a month they had both reached two kilos and went home full time for the mother to care for them. The sister told me there was only one placenta so they felt they were a gift from God. (February 1996)

I was pleased when the twins I had been feeding came to see me. The littler one is still smaller but they are growing and are now five months old. I am still giving the mother extra peanuts to supplement her diet and produce milk for them both.

18. The Tokuni

We are excited at what the Lord is doing amongst the Tokuni people in the lowlands south west of Korupun.

The advance and embrace of Christianity by Papuan tribes' people was complex. On first contact evangelists often met resistance, were threatened, attacked and actively discouraged. In general National evangelists from the same or similar cultures had greater success than the expatriate missionaries. Unravelling the thoughts, motivations and agendas of individuals and groups within a clan was always difficult. Sometimes evangelists found whole communities ready for them and eager to learn more about the new ways. Shortly before her retirement Jessie was in Taiyeve in the Lakes Plain to teach a health workers course. While there, Moses, one of their Bible School students, returned home for a vacation.

He has a real desire to reach out to the lost. He had heard about a tribe further east towards the mountains who were unreached. When he and his friends came to the last village before the foothills they stopped and slept there. As they moved on next morning the villagers ran after them and refused to let them go any further. They explained that maybe the people he was searching for were unfriendly, why not just sit in their village and teach them about this new way. They forced them to stay. (September 2000)

Nor was it unusual for tribes who originally reacted strongly and violently against the coming of Christian evangelists to later welcome them into their homes and villages. Such was the case with the tribe known generally as the Tokuni people, though the tribe call themselves the Dajup Kaga (bamboo people) or also Kop Kaga (lowland people). Their conversion to Christianity makes an interesting case study on the hit and miss nature of missionary work, the personal risks faced by evangelists and the benefits of perseverance.

Les Henson (a missionary colleague) had tried on several occasions to reach this tribe and had been rebuffed. When he finally made contact, they were threatened with bows and arrows when they neared the village and had returned home disappointed.

Les Henson believes the Tokuni originally rejected his overtures because they knew he lived and worked among the Momina people, their traditional enemies.

'Both groups frequently raided each other and stole women and children, while killing the men,' Les said. 'I first made contact with the Tokuni when I carried out a helicopter survey in 1978, about a year before I moved into Sumo to live among the Momina.'

Also on board the helicopter were Les' colleagues Bruce Maclean and Jim Yost. The helicopter landed on the river bank about 150 metres from a longhouse where people lived. Les recalls the events:

'We walked through the water and then took a short path towards the longhouse. We were greeted by a group of agitated women and children who vigorously indicated that we should leave. Erring on the side of caution we made our way back to the riverbank. On the other side of the river was a group of about 15 hostile men waving their bows and arrows in a threatening manner. Recognising that the threat was real we decided it was wiser to make a quick exit. My time over the next 10 years was largely spent reaching out to the various Momina villages. In the late 1980s I made another attempt to survey the Tokuni area by helicopter, but despite landing at what I believed were Tokuni villages, no people were present. It was not until 1994 that we began to have some friendly contact with the Tokuni through our farthest Momina village to the east.'

Les and his wife Wapke left West Papua in December 1995 but by then the ever-persistent evangelists were again working with the Tokuni.

Because they have now seen what a difference it has made in the tribes in the north, east and west of them they want to know what the message is about. They invited some of the church leaders from the Wamena church plus a clinic worker to go in and teach them. They were welcomed back the second time and given gifts from the people with the request for a permanent evangelist to teach them. Pray for the right man to be chosen. Pray for those going into this area as four of the team went down with cerebral malaria after they got back to Wamena. It will not be an easy area to work in, plus the people are nomadic and are moving around. (May 1996)

Kevin and Allyson Martin accepted the challenge of serving among the Tokuni. Kevin provides more detail on how the 'bamboo people' began the journey towards Christianity:

'I joined a National friend and colleague, Otto Kobak (now deceased) in visiting the Tokuni area on numerous occasions beginning in 1995. I think what made it a successful engagement was that the people were ready to receive an outside influence by this time whereas with Les and his colleagues they were very fearful of the outside world, although at one point Allyson and I were confronted with hostility during a linguistic survey. At one village we tried to land in by helicopter we were shot at with arrows. This also was out of fear and ignorance of what we had to offer. Those who were accepting of us had come to see the benefit of healthcare, modern education, and our message of the Gospel. In October 1997, under Otto's leadership, the National church sent a health worker, his family and a young evangelist by the name of Demet Pahabol. Less than a year later we began milling wood for our house but did not move to Tokuni as a family until September 1999.'

The Tokuni

We are praising the Lord that a Peace Ceremony is about to take place in the Southern Lowlands at Tokuni next week. This is a momentous occasion when three long standing enemy chiefs come together to make a peace agreement so they can all listen to the Gospel safely....Amazing as it may seem many of the tribes have always used blood as part of their appeasement to the spirits, cure for sickness and evoking curses onto unsuspecting people. Therefore it is not such a strange thing to them to find that Jesus shed his blood for their sins. The strange part to them is that it is free, and they do not have to work for it and pay for it, just receive it with no strings attached. Very little is a free gift in this society. There is always a hidden string attached somewhere. (March 1999)

19. Church and state

At the moment things are all up in the air here. John (Wilson) *called last week on the radio to say my work permit had still not come through and it is not through by the end of the month I will have to leave.* (July 1986)

The island of New Guinea is divided into two roughly equal parts, the former Dutch territory, West Papua, to the west; a former Australian mandated territory of Papua New Guinea to the east. During the first half of the twentieth century far more of Papua New Guinea was explored, fossicked, settled, planted and fought over than in the western region though great tracts of highland wilderness on both sides of the border remained ignorant of the outside world as it remained ignorant of them.

Australia's knowledge and interest in Papua New Guinea was greatly elevated during World War Two. Thousands of Australian servicemen fought the Japanese there and many died. Wartime newsreels and war photographers showed pictures of the 'fuzzy wuzzy angels', native stretcher bearers helping bring badly wounded Australians down the wet, slippery and dangerous slopes of the Kokoda track where a small band of young, ill-trained Australian servicemen confronted and, after fierce fighting, halted the Japanese advance. Many of these servicemen returned home with an enduring sense of gratitude and concern for Papuan Nationals and this further fuelled a post-war zeal to modernise the country.

By the mid-1950s the same zeal was at work in the western half of the island but there was a marked contrast in approach. In the east the separation of church and state was more clearly delineated than in the west. In *Torn Between Two Worlds,* Australian historian and former missionary Margaret Reeson reconstructed the arrival of the outside world in the Mendi Valley of Papua New Guinea in October 1950. She astutely recorded the reaction of local people to the intrusion.

> "Have you seen the other group across the river?" enquired another observer. "No? There seem to be two sorts of *mbali,* white ones. One clan is called Government and the other is called Mission. The Government clan appears to be very strong and they have many brown men working for them. They seem to be the lawmakers, the judges, the powerful ones. The Mission on the other hand know about ritual and magic and has contact with the spirits. Both clans seem to be very rich and possess many remarkable things. Which group ought we to follow to bring the maximum wealth and success to ourselves?"

By contrast, no such delineation existed in West Papua. The cash strapped and poorly resourced Dutch government had outsourced much of the responsibility for servicing the western part of the island to the missions. It was a deliberate policy and it was the missions, not the government that built airstrips, organised air services, brought in supplies, erected makeshift hospitals and schools and arranged for the medical and educational needs of its people

In *God's Invasion* Robert Wick records that '…the Dutch officials were most enthusiastic about the work of the missionaries.'

He attributed the following comments to the then Director of the Bureau of Native Affairs for Netherlands New Guinea, Dr deBruyn:

> 'Before the boons of civilization can be brought to Stone Age natives, a revolution in their mental attitude has to be effected. That's what Christian missionaries are dramatically accomplishing…. These missionaries know far more about this part of New Guinea and its people than does the government. We are glad to follow their lead.'

Robert Wick says the Dutch authorities were so impressed with the progress missionaries were making they even allowed some missionary wives to enter the Baliem Valley months before a government post was established there.

In some ways little changed when authority was transferred from the Dutch to Indonesia in 1963. The missions still bore the brunt of responsibility for providing services in the highlands. They continued to press into new and unreached regions well ahead of the government, opening up the frontiers to Christianity and western influence. What changed most with the transition from Dutch to Indonesian control was the official attitude to the missions. The government controlled visas and its Indonesian bureaucrats were ever ready to exercise that control. It was the ban on missionary visas that originally frustrated Jessie's efforts to work in West Papua. It was only after the failed 30 September communist coup in 1965 that her visa finally came through. Visa issues and work permits were a recurring theme in Jessie's life and letters and a recurring concern for all missionaries working in the province.

Some of you have probably heard ... that there is a big problem regarding my work permit renewal. In July I was given 10 days to leave the country. When the people heard the news I might have to leave they were very upset and all the churches began to pray. You can imagine how excited they all were when the papers finally came through with four days to the deadline. The Government has a policy now that 10 years should be sufficient for missionaries to accomplish their work and I have had twice that amount. (September 1986)

Bureaucratic demands intruded into many aspects of mission life.

We have just heard that there are new regulations ... and we now have to have our station name painted on something so that a plane flying overhead can see it. Letters have to be two metres long. So Elinor has had fun trying to get someone to do it. (March 1985)

But visas and permits were the most constant irritant.

I hoped to give you more definite word regarding my furlough plans by now, but the wheels of government offices grind slowly, especially in the election year. My work permit has still not returned from Jakarta. In the meanwhile we have had some startling news that 14 of our missionaries have had their visas cancelled. (March 1987)

We are praising the Lord for my work permit which arrived two weeks ago. But because of the new regulations we now have to wait five weeks before we can leave…. We are thrilled that other crises regarding visas for us have been settled for the time being. Irian Jaya has been ruled a special area, needing missionaries. (June 1987).

Last week my extension came through. Unexpectedly my work permit also came through. For the past 10 years my work permit has always been six months late. Now I had two options and I had to decide what to do. Either leave with my extension that week or wait another month for my work permit to be processed. So far none of the missionaries who had their papers stamped 'non-renewable' have had to leave and a number have had their visas renewed. Please continue to pray that the Lord will overrule in this situation. (January 1988)

The elections went off here without any incidents, but of course the votes are still not completely counted. Do pray for the future of this country. On my return, I heard that there had been another government edict regarding visas for pilots and nurses. Those who have been here for more than five years could lose their visa next year. This will include Sue and myself, plus a lot of senior MAF pilots. MAF is hoping to get an audience with the governor and appeal. (August 1999)

So much had changed since Jessie first touched down in West Papua in 1966, but sometimes it seemed much remained the same.

There is still no word on the renewal of our visas. So I guess no news is good news. Keep praying for the situation. We are praising the Lord that even though the pilots have lost their visas they have been able to get new ones almost immediately. But we have heard that one of the Dutch missions has lost a number of visas with no new ones being available. (March 2000)

20. To baptise or not to baptise

It has been a time of real rejoicing in these last few weeks as several of the churches have had baptisms.

Baptism is a fundamental rite of the Christian church, yet it caused much soul-searching among the missionaries of West Papua. How much knowledge, training and understanding should Nationals have of Christianity before they were accepted for baptism? Were they fully aware what it meant to be a Christian? How much of the traditional religions, superstitions and practices could be retained while still professing to be a Christian? These were all vexing questions and the different missions and missionaries often reached different answers to the common problems.

We have seen the clash of cultures elsewhere in Jessie's writings. It had a direct impact on her own medical work. Time and time again local people shied away from western medicine that could cure them in favour of traditional medicine, local practices, beliefs and customs – often with deadly consequences. Traditional justice, payback and family responsibilities were other issues that also weighed heavily on the lives and consciences of newly-Christian people. Christian conversion and baptism also divided communities.

Some men from another area tried to interrupt and disrupt a service. Why, we don't know, but we assume that they had relatives that were being baptised and they didn't approve. The service continued in an orderly way despite threats and insolence from the armed and feathered men. Do pray for these men from the Lugwa, who are so much against the Gospel, and also for these newly baptised believers that they may not be intimidated in any way but may stay firm to the Lord. The people of Lugwa are just three days walk away from here and are related to the Grand Valley Dani folk who are very much opposed to the Gospel, mainly because their chiefs have forbidden them to listen in case they lose control over their people. (April 1971)

To baptise or not to baptise was a question that was never fully resolved during Jessie's time in West Papua. These excerpts from her letters show the tension and anxiety that so often accompanied the ritual of baptism among the Kimyal and other West Papuan communities.

In March there will be baptisms in two of our more distant villages, two to three days walk. We are hoping to go by helicopter as I am sure I will conk out half way. We will stay overnight to attend the feast and then the baptisms the following day. Approximately 50 people will be baptised. Do pray for the participants as they publicly announce their faith in the Lord and their complete break from the evil spirits. This is a very special day for them and a big decision to completely trust the Lord. Many of these outer areas are still very active in their spirit worship. (March 1986)

We were greatly encouraged in July when 50 people from Korupun and nearby villages were baptised. It has been a long time since anyone from here was baptised because in the past there was a lot of misunderstanding about baptism. Some thought you couldn't be a Christian unless you were baptised. After much prayer and discussion the pastor decided that they would make people wait until they showed by their lives and actions that they were different and that everyone knew that they were changed. (October 1991)

Baptism though, is central to the Christian message, and a cause for celebration among most Christian communities. So it was in Korupun when church elders agreed to a mass baptism. Jessie joined the celebration and later shared the colour, excitement and sense of ceremony with her prayer network.

The shouting and the tumult have died down since all the people have returned home after the excitement of the long awaited baptisms. Pre-baptism fever coloured everything for days before the event.

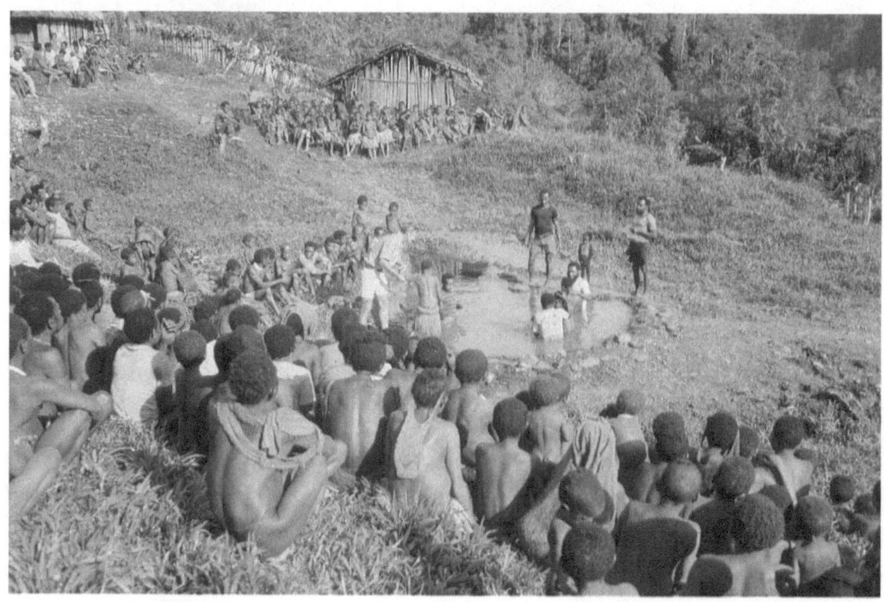

All the candidates had to be questioned re their faith and when they accepted the Lord. Some became very nervous and ran away. With 214 people to be checked, it took some time for the elders from the four churches involved to sift through them all. For various reasons it must be nearly 10 years since they had a baptism right here in Korupun. The day before the actual baptisms they had a big celebration feast. At least 2000 people were present. All the wood and hundreds of rocks had to be gathered and brought to the feasting place the day before in readiness for an early start the next morning (4 am). A pond had to be dug and prepared in a little stream nearby. All this was done to the accompaniment of singing, chanting and shouting. The singing went on through most of the night.

We were woken before dawn on the feast day. The hillside was like an anthill. Everyone had a job to do, some bringing in the grass, ferns and banana leaves to line the food pits, while others dig the pits and cut up pigs; the women to make blood and sausages from the intestines; the men to build frames to hold the wood where the rocks would rest, while the fire heats them up underneath. Such a bountiful supply of food.

Most of the clinic workers walked in (from their villages). The trails are very dangerous at present because of the heavy rains. My house was like Grand Central Station with everyone coming in to talk, drink tea and eat biscuits, replace their medicine supplies and enjoy the company of others. One of my midwives braved the slippery trail. She was excited to see me. It must be 12 months since I last saw her. I was warmly welcomed, hugged and chucked under the chin. In the midst of all this, the helicopter came in and out several times taking supplies to some of our far away villages where we are building new clinics. All in all it was organised chaos.

The day dawned bright and clear – in fact a little too bright as we all got sunburnt after sitting for hours in the hot sun. The church leaders had done a wonderful job of organising the whole day. They had all the participants in line and numbered. Each person was called by name when their turn came as were the elders who would baptise them. Hours of work behind the scenes. The pastor gave an excellent word on what the valley here was like before the Gospel came and what a change had come since the people have turned to the Lord and stopped fighting and practising witchcraft.

Seven elders, including Orin, were in the water at the one time. Because the water was so cold they alternated every 15 minutes with other groups of men. It was exciting to see some really old people taking part along with a good mixture of all ages. In between each group being baptised about 10 teenagers sang along with their guitars. After the ceremony was over, all the newly baptised folk, plus all the other baptised believers had a communion service together on the airstrip. That swelled the group to about 700 which is nearly 50 per cent of the population of the valley here.
(March 1999)

The Bible records many of the conflicts and divisions of the early Christian Church. Not surprising then that human feelings and frailties also came into play in the Papuan highlands.

During the last six months one of the close-by villages decided they would break-off from the main Korupun Church. They had sent several young men out to Bible School (who were not recommended by the church) and when they returned they were very unhappy because they were not given the job of pastor, amongst other grievances. Pray for the village of Maningmog, and particularly those who wish to split the church. This is our most heathen village, where most of the relatives of an old witch doctor live. Do pray for this conflict and that the elders will have wisdom to deal with it.

A couple of weeks ago, in this same village (Maningmog) a woman delivered a baby at 3 am one morning. She had a haemorrhage and died. They didn't call me, which is sad, but I guess it was all of a sudden. The baby was doing fine until someone in the village had a dream that the mother came back and asked why they were feeding her baby. She said it belonged to her and she had come back for it. They stopped feeding it and he died. I was upset. The Lord reminded me that it is His church and He is building it. We are just the caretakers. (October 1999)

21. Aches, pains and emergencies

February and the nut season has started again. February, March are very busy for the clinic with many accidents from machetes and falls from fragile branches.

I had a call to come down to the clinic, this fellow had been climbing the tree to cut off the large nuts when he fell on his head, dripping blood he covered his head with a banana leaf and walked an hour to the clinic. His skull was split wide open, broken nose and numerous cuts and bruises. I stitched him up and asked if he had pain and he said, 'just a slight headache!' I guess they have hard skulls and are tough.

As the only qualified medical worker in Korupun Jessie dealt with the full range of health needs, from primary health care for babies and breast feeding mothers to the more dramatic accidents, health problems and medical emergencies that were part and parcel of highland life.

Elinor and I went off to one of our furthest villages last week by helicopter. I had a clinic for all those who needed it and then gave the injections for those with goitre problems. The high rainfall here washes the iodine out of the soil and this causes deficient children (cretins) so an injection every four years can stop this. We had eight inches of rain in the past two days.
(August 1980)

Last week they brought a little two-year-old into the clinic who had a very bad burn on his foot. It was a very strange place so I asked what had happened. Apparently the little sister who was looking after him whilst the mother was in the gardens got exasperated with him because he kept getting into mischief and wouldn't do what she said, so to teach him a lesson in behaviour she dumped him in the fire. (January 1982)

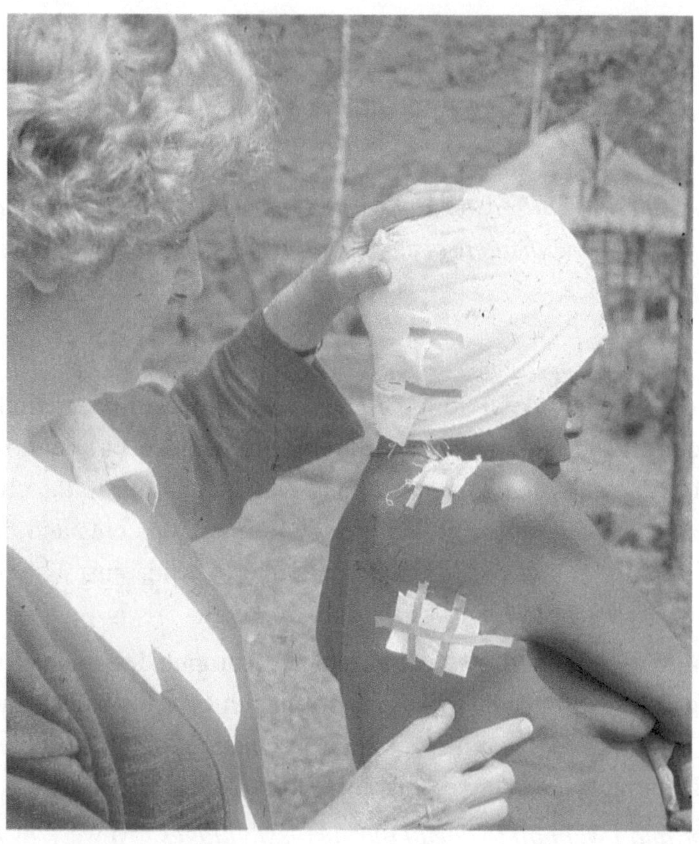

This afternoon a fellow walked for two hours from the next valley. He had chopped off his thumb. In spite of a makeshift bandage he had haemorrhaged badly and was very weak. I was amazed he had managed to walk so far. He even brought the thumb but the time lapse was too great so I pulled the skin across to stop the bleeding but think it will take a long time to heal.

Another fellow had split his big toe down the centre. It required a lot of suturing but he will not stop walking on it!

Yesterday the people came rushing up to tell me they were carrying in a girl who had fallen the night before. Apparently she had been out helping her father trap possums in the moonlight. They didn't miss her for two hours. Then the older sister had a dream that her sister had had an accident. She woke up and went looking for her. They found she had fallen off the path on the edge of the river, head first into some rocks. When they picked her up they thought she was dead. They carried her back to the house and the father started praying for her. When they realised she was alive they carried her in for seven hours. She was not responding well. We called the doctor but he thought just observe her. Orin Kidd and the pastor came and prayed over her and her family prayed all night. This morning she is much better, a miracle as she had fallen at least 10 feet onto her head!

This past week the Government gave me a lot of deworming pills so I decided to dose everyone up at the same time. The worms cause malnutrition and respiratory problems. So hopefully it will help. We went from village to village and treated more than 1000 people.

I have been tube feeding premature babies too tired to suck, three-hourly. The mothers bring them to me. Last night one mother came knocking on my door saying the baby was choking and couldn't breathe. He had inhaled some vomit. I sucked out what I could, quickly did some artificial respiration, gave some adrenaline and an inhalation and he started to improve and is now doing fine again. She curled up on my lounge room floor for the night. Then we all got a bit of sleep. (1986)

This past week Dr David Gee came to visit the Kidds. I was glad when he offered to amputate the toe of a man who had been bitten by a centipede and was beginning to go gangrene. (I wasn't looking forward to doing it). The smell was very high. The men in his hut told him to go and live in the forest because of the smell. He was delighted to be rid of his toe. A few days later I did some skin grafts on the stump.

One morning I woke up to hear a lady wailing on my front door step. She told me her child was close to death as he was badly burnt. I went down to the village to check it out and sure enough there was a 10 year-old boy crouched by his hut. Apparently he and two of his friends had been out on the mountain hunting possums. They were sleeping in an old draughty garden house. Because it was very cold they built a big fire and went off to sleep. They woke up to find a blazing roof caving in on them. Two had minor burns but one was a real mess from his head to his waist on the left side. It took us an hour each day to do his dressing. (August 1995)

This week they spent six days carrying a 15 year-old girl in obstructed labour over the trail using a rice bag secured at each corner with a pole. Ten men took it in turns to carry her over the mountain. We all prayed for the rain to hold off, which it did for about five minutes and then it bucketed down. By then it was too late for a plane and as I sedated her I was afraid she would rupture her uterus. We spoke to the doctor at 7am and they were able to divert a plane to pick her up. We hear she had an assisted delivery but the baby was dead. Fortunately the girl is OK but will no doubt take some time to recover. These emergencies are exhausting. (1996)

A little kid arrived at the door and said they had carried a lass from the next valley on a stretcher. She had had a baby three weeks ago and the placenta (after birth) had not come. She was given penicillin but that was not sufficient so she started to bleed, and they thought she would die. She was so anaemic she really needed a blood transfusion. After some medication she stopped bleeding, so hopefully we can get her back on her feet. She is just a young girl and the baby is doing fine. I checked her this evening and she is improving for which I am thankful. (February 2000)

22. The 'death' month

The people call August the 'death' month because so many babies die of the flu.

The ever increasing contact with the outside world and more regular movement of people around the highlands greatly increased the risk of infectious diseases and epidemics. But the arrival of the missionaries also brought with it modern means to combat such diseases and for the first time in the highlands, people had some defence against infection. Immunisation programs were always a priority because vaccinations changed the dynamics in the battle against infectious diseases.

The science of vaccinations has been known and accepted since 1796 when Edward Jenner famously used cowpox to inoculate against the deadly smallpox disease. From there science made slow but inevitable progress driven by inquiring minds and the desire to ease human suffering. In 1914 a vaccine was developed to protect against pertussis, a disease more commonly known as whooping cough. In 1926 diphtheria joined the list of preventable diseases, followed in 1938 by tetanus. After World War Two these three vaccines were combined and given as the DPT vaccine – what is now better known as Triple Antigen. Pharmaceuticals were being produced on an industrial scale thanks to technical advances. Costs fell, making them readily available, and vaccinations were progressively developed for a range of other common diseases like measles, mumps and rubella. Few services Jessie provided during her 35 years as a missionary nurse saved as many lives and prevented suffering as much as the vaccination programs she organised and administered.

Trying to set up a DPT clinic in a village is easier said than done. The Korupun area has never had a campaign of any kind for its babies. So there was much interest and speculation about it all. In one village we used the school building, in another a central place in the village and in another a flat rock where we could put things out of the mud. Everywhere we went there were milling, sweating bodies wanting to see everything. Kids elbowed their way to the front so they wouldn't miss a thing. No one left till all the babies had been vaccinated because they wanted to see whose babies cried and whose were brave and which ones kicked and screamed to get away. Fathers, grandmothers, aunts and uncles all sharing in the excitement, peering in windows and standing on rocks to get a better view.

As I left Korupun to go to the mountains the people said to me to be careful as the people up there are all making bows and arrows and a war could be breaking out anytime. Be ready to duck. In spite of a threatening war between the two villages all the ladies and their babies in the village turned out in full force. The four and five year olds were disappointed because they couldn't get a needle or should I say their parents were disappointed. Several times I had to move a black woolly head out of my way so I could see to put the needle on the syringe as some little kid was peering into my pot of needles. I almost injected the wrong child when one stepped in front of me as I was about to give a shot. Another knocked the syringe out of my hand as they tried to get close as possible to see how I did it. All in a day's work! Needles to them are something special.

We have heard that there is whooping cough in the next village. I am trying to get as many babies as possible started on their course. A real miracle that the vaccine was available and we had the connections to get it into the interior right away. We will try to arrange for the helicopter to get us out to some of the more distant villages as soon as possible.

Speaking of injections makes me remember one old man who came to the clinic with a tooth abscess and a very swollen jaw. When I told him to turn around to give him a shot of penicillin, he very crossly informed me that he didn't have a pain in his bottom, it was his tooth and he wanted the shot there. I guess he thought I was very dumb. (August 1981)

Recently a girl said to me that 'the month of death' was here again. She had her child clasped in her arms as if to defy any sickness to 'hit' her child. Looking back I see what was meant by that statement. It seemed that during the months of August and September each year there is an epidemic of some kind leaving a trail of death and sadness in its wake. This year it has been a very bad flu epidemic where practically all the children between one and 14 years have had it in one form or another. They stagger into clinic with red glassy eyes and a temperature over 102 degrees. They are immediately given a bucket bath to try and reduce the temperature and fever (wearing no clothes does have its advantages). After they are dried off they receive their lemon juice, soup and medication. Some mornings we have had over 100 children through the clinic and have used up to 1000 aspirins in a week.

The afternoons see a never ending procession of people to my door to receive their soup rations. Most of these children stop eating and drinking when they are sick so the soup is a bribe to keep them hydrated. I have certainly made gallons of soup over the past month and I think I could receive a diploma in soup making. This afternoon a mother came to the door with her child clasped in her arms. Unfortunately there was nothing I could do as the child was already dead. I was trying to comfort the mother when she said: 'It isn't your fault. It's God's business and He has taken my child to heaven. He knows best.' Do pray for these people in the harshness of their land and the constant loss of their beloved children. Do pray too for the clinic workers as they try to cope with so many ill children. There have been 12 deaths in the next valley. (September 1985)

In 1986 Sue Trenier and Jessie combined with various clinic workers on an extended vaccination trip around Lolat.

We went by helicopter divided into four teams and all walked in different directions. Some walked for three days, some two days and Sue and I walked to the closer villages, three hours there and three hours back. It was very steep, wet and slippery. They were all laughing because I was so slow! We had to climb up from the river to the heli-pad. The boys had to pull me over the big rocks as my shoes would not grip. We got home just on dark as it started to pour with rain. We vaccinated 63 children for TB. In all we did 400 children for DPT, polio and measles. We gave out Vitamin A to the kids over 12 months. [I was aching all over]. When we got back the people had prepared a feast for us to say thank-you, we were embarrassed because they can't really spare the pigs but we couldn't refuse.

Sue Trenier has fond and vivid memories of these expeditions, often working with teams of Nationals from the Eastern Highland's church district to train medical workers and run immunisation programs:

'There was a period when Jessie and I were doing quite a lot of village work together, not only in the Kimyal or Hupla areas where we served but also in Yali and Momina areas. Early on I found out what a great thing it was to have Jessie with us on the team!!! This one time the pair of us were sleeping in a small school building, our sleeping bags squeezed in. She would leave the organising part to me to get the people gathered, get the workers in teams etc. and she would join in the activities and the training. She would disappear though after a bit, and to our amazement, when we returned to our habitat, she would have prepared the most amazingly interesting snack/lunch or whatever. She might have cheese and biscuits and coffee, or cuppa soup (so welcome in those cold mountain areas), a bar of chocolate or special 'something'. How she did it I do not know, but that always revived us. These treats all came in the endless packets/parcels which her wonderful supporters sent her regularly.'

Mothers seemed to understand, almost instinctively, that the new medicine could achieve what local custom could not, and protect their children from harm, even if the highland children, like children everywhere, were less sure.

'Don't be afraid, it's only the healing lady. She won't hurt you,' were words that were often repeated this week to uplifted, tearful faces as I continued to give the second series of DPT injections against whooping

cough to the children. Whooping cough is a mean killer up here and there seems to be an epidemic every four years. I like to keep a jump ahead if the vaccine is available. Not everyone will cooperate unfortunately, but the people are learning to trust us more and more and they prefer needles to any other kind of medication. Every morning we have a roll up of about 140 children. I would have been glad of some earplugs as most of the kids didn't agree with their mothers that the 'wesena gel' didn't hurt. (March 1986)

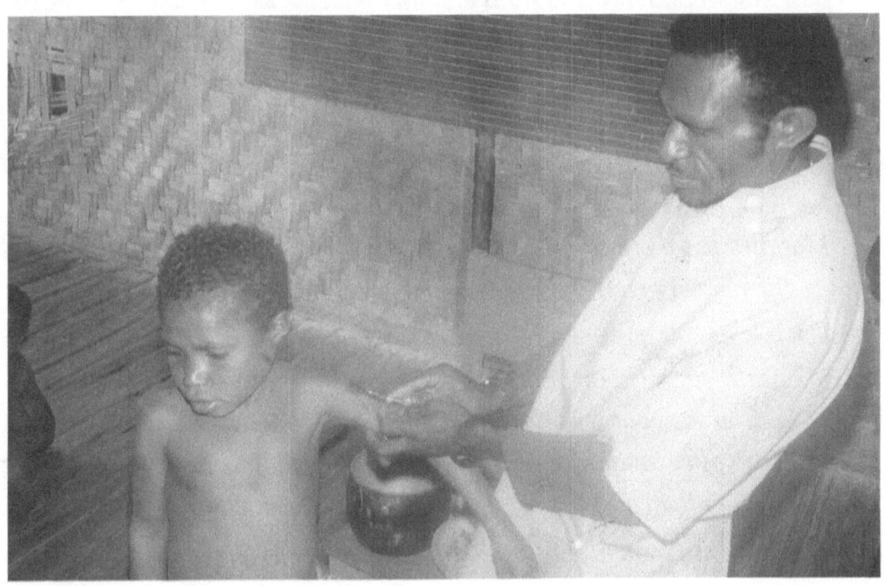

I came back to Korupun to find a virulent type of flu raging, which knocked the whole population down. It wasn't just flu, but all kinds of complications that set in afterwards that really laid people low. The clinic was a hive of industry with a trail of woebegone people passing through. I made up gallons of soup to give to the people who had stopped eating, to try and keep them drinking. We all had our turn of being laid low with it. There have been six deaths in our outlying areas where they didn't come in for treatment. The Swart Valley was really hard hit with over 60 deaths among the Dani population. (March 1987)

Last week they brought me a little three-day-old baby with a bad case of pneumonia. That afternoon it stopped breathing so I quickly did mouth to mouth resuscitation, artificial respirator, stimulants and a lot of prayer. It finally started to breathe again and is now doing just fine for such a little strap of a baby. I have also started using gum leaves in boiling water as an inhalation and it works very well. (May 1989)

The whole population has been laid low with it (flu) and we have had a busy clinic for weeks. The worst is over but we're now starting to get complications that follow in its wake. We have used over 15,000 aspirin this past month and now the flu is steadily making its way to our outposts. We have not had a death here thus far. One evening, just on dusk, a boy came to tell me that there was a baby who was near death in one of our villages. I knew it would be dark by the time I got home so I put a torch in my pocket and set off up the mountain. I was thankful to get there in the last of the daylight. I was glad I had gone as the baby had viral meningitis which often follows the flu. I slipped and slithered down the muddy waterlogged path in the pouring rain. I was absolutely drenched.

Each morning it is quite a sight to see 10 babies and their mothers sitting in two circles on the floor of the clinic all covered with sheets. The inhalation pots sit in the centre of the circles whilst the babies breathe or scream in the eucalyptus inhalation. The noise is deafening, like a lot of lambs separated from their mothers all yelling at once. (September 1989)

'Yetty, will you look at this child, and this one and this one? Whatever is the matter with them? Their faces are all swollen.' For the first time ever, we suddenly had an epidemic of mumps in the valley. Children looking like chipmunks and adults looking as if they had suddenly gained 10 kilos with their round faces. No one was really ill, just miserable. (October 1991)

I was woken at 3 am by someone pounding on the door. 'Yonas's little three-year-old was desperately ill. Could I come?' I hastily pulled on a track suit, grabbed my emergency bag and off into the night. Sadly, by the time we got there she had already died. It appears to be a virulent type of gastro-enteritis – healthy one day and gone the next. Another little one died last night which is so sad. We have heard on radio that 20 people have died at Lolat (two days walk from here).

The 'death' month

We were really sad about Yonas's little girl. (He did my washing and does radio). The whole village mourned for her and before the funeral the village cooked potatoes to give to everyone who came. A special honour. Sijeit preached. They kept the body two days which was unusual – so everyone could see her and the mourning went on day and night. Sijeit started his message by saying the night before he had a dream. That he was walking with this little girl along the trail when suddenly she started to drift into the air like soap bubbles you make from children's ring bubble maker. He stood watching her disappear and then a voice said, 'Don't wait for her to return to you, she has come into heaven with me. Don't cry. She is happy.'

In between all this a 15 year-old unmarried girl delivered a baby. No one knew she was pregnant (amazing in this culture). That almost sparked off a war except for the cool head and handling of one of the fathers involved. Pig payments had to be paid to the girl's family.

Life, births, deaths, marriages and problems go on as it does everywhere. (January 1995)

Bit by bit, government services came to the highlands, supplementing, complementing and occasionally displacing the work of the mission public health programs.

We were all called out to a government seminar in Wamena for the WATCH Program which is 'Women and their Children's Health Project'. This program has introduced rabbits, chickens, fish etc. to the area to try and upgrade the health of the women. Unfortunately the men have taken most of it over and it hasn't really helped the women. However they are trying. (May 1995)

Whilst she (Beatrix Watofa, an Irianese mission candidate) *was here she upgraded two workers on the microscope. They checked over 450 specimens. Now we are busy giving out medications for all the parasites she found. Very few people had negative results so we trust they are healthier (including me) now they are not feeding so many inside friends.* (February 1996)

23. Translating the Bible

Many Dani folk ask for work so they can buy a small portion of scripture translated for them, and stencilled off. This is a slow and expensive task for us but the joy in the faces of these folk as they read it is worth it all.

The written word is such a routine part of everyday life that we tend to take it for granted. But words, particularly written words, have a power about them, a power that many West Papuan Nationals quickly recognised with the coming of the missionaries and the black, leather-bound books they carried, read, pondered and prayed over. By the time Jessie first touched down at Karubaga translators were already busily working on selected verses of the Bible to share with their Dani converts – though a full translation of the Bible was still many years off. To many Dani the words the missionaries spoke had magic about them, magic they were eager to learn and understand, and this magic was embodied in their written words.

Akkenok is sitting by the stove reading his 'Kywone' or 'Living words' which is what they call the scriptures. He has made a cover out of some cardboard. They are only duplicated copies so are very precious....These folk have very little translated for them and what they have they love and memorise and tell it to others. (1967)

The only schools in remote parts of West Papua at this time were mission schools. They identified the best, brightest and most promising students they could find and set them on an express pathway of learning, including enrolment at Bible school. The Bible school students were destined to play a big role in the life of the young church, but more than that, they would become the new intelligentsia – the first tentative links between old faiths and new religion, tribal traditions and the modern world. Little wonder that their graduation was the cause of great excitement.

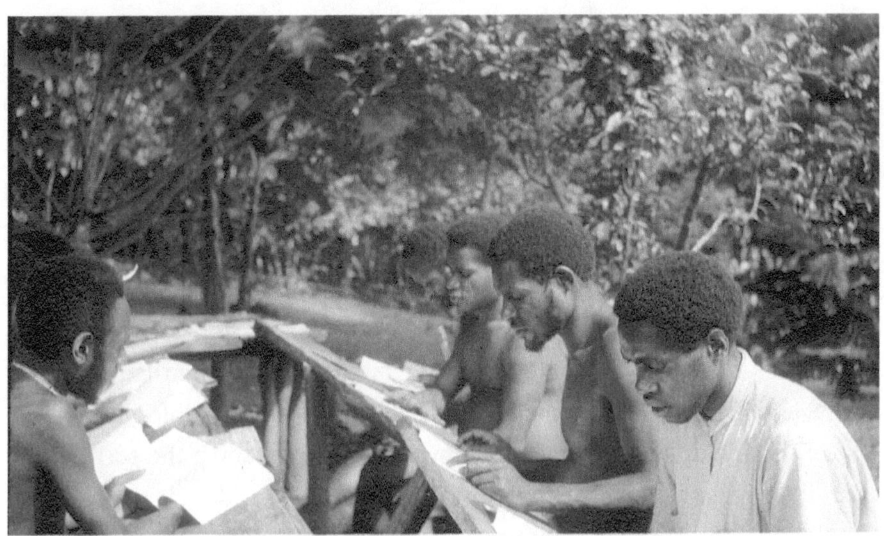

Everyone was in a fever of excitement. Graduation was looming. The very first graduation of our Bible School students who have studied for three years was about to take place. They will then move back to their own villages and communities to be a help and encouragement to their elders and pastors. (May 1968)

In this multi-skilled vocation everyone had a role to play in every aspect of mission life, including Jessie.

I have been helping out in the examination of the graduates from our literacy schools. We have 20 schools here at Karubaga. When each class has finished the 12th primer they are examined to see if they have learnt well. They are then given a diploma if they pass the test. Much encouragement is needed for these shaking students as they wait their turn to be examined. By keeping a close eye on the graduating students we are able to keep a high standard in all our schools. Some of them have memorised all the books and can fool their teachers, but when it comes to an exam they are lost if it is not well learnt. (February 1972)

Dani is just one of more than 250 languages spoken in Papua. Every time missionaries encroached on a new area or reached new people the process of communicating, teaching literacy, and translating the Bible and other texts began anew. Indonesian was the official language; English was the first language of most new missionaries while each tribal group had its own language and a smattering of other nearby languages and dialects to allow communication with their neighbours. It was a linguistic melting pot.

The core skills set out in this position description taken from the World Team website in 2016 could have equally applied to missionaries entering unreached parts of West Papua half a century earlier.

'Use your translation skills to help deliver the scriptures to people in a language and form they can understand. Many tribal languages are unwritten, leaving entire people groups with no Bible they can read. You can help people grow in faith as they receive the scripture in their heart language. Plus you'll have the joy of developing deep relationships with national translators you work with. You may also help develop literacy programs or serve as a translation consultant and advisor.'

In 1980 when Jessie moved to Korupun she was asked to supervise the literacy program there.

In June I will be attending a Literacy Workshop to help me teach the Kimyal people to read and write in their own language. Because of the change in the Indonesian cathography (alphabet) we are having to change quite a few letters in the Kimyal alphabet to make it as close as possible to the Indonesian. The Christians are very keen to learn, especially as Elinor gets more and more of the scriptures translated. There was great excite-ment a few weeks ago when she finished the book of Titus and gave it to the people. The elders have been begging for more scriptures as they said they knew by heart all that had been translated and they needed something new to share with the people. Because their way of life and thought patterns are so different to ours it is important that they learn what the scriptures say regarding certain matters and that they learn to make their own decisions in the light of it and not just accept what we say as final. (June 1980)

We are praising the Lord that we have the rough draft of our new primers (books to teach the people to read and write) finished. Hopefully in the next couple of weeks we will be able to get the stencils cut and a trial number given out to teachers. (August 1981)

Jessie's experiences with the Kimyal language were no doubt similar to those of her colleagues Kathryn and Paul Kline who began working among the Kimyal in 1969. One of the first tasks of any missionary working in a new area among new people was to learn the local languages. The task could be as complex as it was necessary. Kathryn Kline shares some of her experiences with the Kimyal language.

'Every language has intonation, the rise and fall of words in a sentence. Some languages are tonal, meaning that words may be spelled in the same way, but carry a different meaning if spoken at a higher or lower pitch. The Kimyal language has a unique structure that is different than English. We have six persons, but Kimyal has nine persons: English has first person singular and plural: I/we, second person singular and plural: you, and third person singular and plural: he/they, but the Kimyal have another category: I/we-two, you-two and he/they-two! Kimyal has the sentence structure with the subject first, then the object, and ending the sentence with the verb or the action word. Concrete thoughts are easy to explain, but subjects such as love, mercy and salvation need to be illustrated.

One must learn their language, and one does not need to be perfect. The Kimyal will always repeat what is being said, and if one listens carefully, they will always say it correctly. Great for language learning! By the time I put my sentence two-thirds together, the Kimyal would give me the rest of the sentence! Also great for language learning!'

The literacy program worked in a similar way to the clinic worker and village midwife programs. It was a train-the-trainer approach with likely candidates selected from the villagers, educated and trained before returning to their village to pass on their knowledge to others. Literacy training and education were intimately connected to Bible study and evangelism. For the missionaries literacy had one primary motivation above all others – to spread the Word.

This past week was a special time for the literacy teachers when they all came to receive their new sets of primers/teaching books for their villages. The bush telegraph worked overtime when the books were ready to be distributed. They all came in for a time of Bible study, receive their supplies of chalk and books and have a feast together. There are 30 teachers so the place was teeming with extra people for a few days as all their friends came along too. Each village has one or two teachers depending on the size of their population. Usually their classes are held each morning at 6 am, after the morning devotions are held in the teaching hut. There is great excitement and motivation to learn to read and write their own language at the moment. Elinor has just had the book of Acts and quite a number of Old Testament stories printed, so there is now more for them to read. Do pray that they will continue to be thrilled to read the Word of God. (June 1987)

Much effort went into Bible translation and landmark events, like the completion of new books, or entire Testaments, were a cause for celebration.

I have just come from a very moving experience when we witnessed the dedication of the Yali New Testament at Ninia. It has taken 17 years to translate and two years for it to be printed, so we are thankful it is finally in the hands of the people. The Yali people organised the whole day themselves which was exciting. They killed 140 pigs for the big feast to feed at least 2000 people, some from four days walk away. John Wilson, the translator, came from Canada especially for the occasion.

Sue, Helen (project Timothy worker) and myself arrived a day earlier to help MAF stagger the flying. Ninia is notorious for its bad weather being 6,600 feet up in the clouds. They were really ambitious as they had planned four landings with VIP guests. We took our sleeping bags and stayed in the original house built by the Dales. The people prayed far into the night for all the preparations for the next day and especially for the weather. They were up again at 3.30 am blowing whistles and banging tins to waken everyone.

The Bible school students sang two new songs they had composed especially for the day. They were followed by a drama organised by Donglu, one of the old witch doctors, depicting when Bruno and Stan walked into the area. The suspicions and the hostile reception they were given by the people – particularly by him and his family. Now he is praising the Lord for the change that came to his own heart and the lives of the people as they have trusted in the Lord and found hope in the future. The proceedings took about four hours. A misty rain started just before the last speech which didn't dampen their spirits, as everyone headed towards the feast to demolish the food set out. (February 1993)

The next year there were similar celebrations at Soba which Jessie again reported in some detail.

Excitement at Soba started to build up two weeks prior to the dedication of the new Bible School Buildings and Hupla New Testament, as village by village they sang and danced their way up the airstrip to bring in the rocks and firewood to be used for the feast to be held after the ceremony. Stepping from the plane, I was greeted by a welcoming committee of men dancing on the airstrip. Bedecked with possum fur hats, decorated with feathers and flowers, bodies bedaubed with red and yellow clay, they were a sight to behold. I had come a week early to help Sue with the last minute preparations for the dedication. Several days before the ceremony the enthusiasm reached a crescendo when Sue and her team of translators were honoured by the people, and were each presented with a large pig. A pig in Hupla land is the ultimate gift. The life of Sue's pig came to an abrupt end after it had escaped for the fifth time and rooted up the vegetable patch. We enjoyed the shared roast pork that night.

'THE DAY' began at 4 am with everyone shouting and pigs squealing as they were hauled off to be slaughtered in the early dawn. The morning dawned clear and bright, but overcast. We were glad for a great day as

we had nine planes and two helicopters landing with government officials. Graham Cousins, the first white missionary to be stationed at Soba, came from the USA especially for the dedication. We were glad of the cloud coverage later on in the day, as we sat with 2000 others on the grass in front of the dais. The people organised the whole day themselves which was quite an accomplishment. They planned a drama including the first two evangelists from Ninia and Tangma who came to explain the Gospel to them. Three times they had to run for their lives with arrows flying around them, before people were ready to listen. The audience sat and listened in rapt attention to the whole program. It was a joy to see the first Hupla New Testament go into the hands of the people, a culmination of 10 years hard work. (July 1994)

Teaching literacy and translating books from the Bible was part of a seemingly never-ending cycle.

Senenob has just been to get some scripture portions to take with him as he does his rounds of all the 38 literacy schools. It takes him over two weeks to do the rounds and check up on everybody. He takes scriptures to sell and chalk for the teachers. He is very faithful which takes a lot of responsibility off me. (January 1995)

We had a translation consultant from the Indonesian Bible Society in here checking the books of John and Romans, which Rosa had translated. He was very happy with the translation and we can now go ahead and print these books. The Bible Society will print the finished New Testament at a much lower cost if one of their consultants has done the checking. The people are excited to be getting some new scriptures to read. We have the privilege of being able to read the whole Bible at any time we like but these people can't do that yet. They appreciate so much more each portion as it is translated. Rosa hopes to come back for two months each year to check what the local translators have done in her absence. (October 1999)

In 2000 the Yali Bible became the first whole Bible to be translated in West Papua. This was Jessie's final year of service in the province. She couldn't disguise her enthusiasm for the project, eagerly reporting on both the preparations and the event itself.

Only eight weeks to go in the countdown to the Yali Bible. Pressure and excitement are mounting as planning meetings and committees have been working overtime to make sure nothing is overlooked for this very special occasion at Ninia. (March 2000)

I wish I could have transported all of you to Ninia for the long awaited dedication of the complete Yali Bible. The day dawned bright and clear. The first plane landed on the airstrip soon after 6 am with important guests, reporters, T.V. cameramen etc. The governor, vice-governor and heads of most government departments including the chief of police and intelligence made an impressive array on the platform which was banked by flowers and ferns.

It was exciting and heart-warming to see the culmination of many years labour. There were many tears shed as the pastors from the different church areas received their copies of the Bible and clasped them tightly in their hands. The Word of the Living God was there in its entirety for them to read at will, the first tribe in Irian Jaya to be able to do so. Praise the Lord for the perseverance of Otto and Luliap during the past nine years as they have worked tirelessly on the Old Testament. The 3000 plus people who attended sat on the hard ground and listened attentively. Some of the older men, dressed in their traditional dress of possum skin hats, feathers, pig tusks and gourds, danced on the airstrip - a good reminder of how far these people have come in 35 years.

The ceremony closed at approximately 2 pm when the Heli Mission helicopter took the governor and his body guards to another airstrip to connect with a larger MAF plane because of the wind curfew at Ninia. We were amazed and delighted that the governor would come to such an occasion in a predominantly Muslim country.

Pray for the Yali people that they will now read their new Bible and not just keep it as a status symbol. The day before the celebration the church had planned a big pig feast and a church dedication at Ballinggama which is approximately one hours walk from Ninia. It was very appropriate that Bruno de Leeuw was able to be there for the occasion as he had been with Stan Dale all those years ago. Ballinggama was the first village where

Bruno preached and the first village where any interest was shown in the Gospel of the Good News that they had brought. Such a change in those hard cannibal hearts to become loving and caring people is something only God could do. (June 2000)

After her retirement Jessie kept tabs on progress in translation, updating her network as news came to hand.

The Dani Old Testament has finally been put into the hands of the Bible Society printers in Java. It has been a long haul for Wesley Dale and the translation team to accomplish this task. Now they are looking to revise the New Testament before it is made into a complete book. (December 2002)

24. Drought, death and desperation

We have had a bad potato shortage for the last six months. The government has promised rice but it hasn't happened. I have a lot of hungry, skinny children at my back door.

Like all subsistence farmers and communities, the Kimyal relied on the elements. Some seasons were good, others not so good and when the rains didn't come or crops failed as they did in 1993, the people suffered.

When the mothers become malnourished they lose their milk to feed their babies. I have bought rice for those who are ill but with 7000 people not much I can do. The last lot of rice that came from Jakarta had rats in the bags, unwelcome visitors who chewed their way out and were chewing at the peoples' leathery feet in the night! They are eagerly awaiting the nut season.

But there were even worse years. In late 1997 Jessie returned to Korupun for her last stint in the high mountains before retirement. She had just completed a long furlough in Australia that included recuperation from a gall bladder operation. The return seemed a bitter parody of the frustrations and difficulties that accompanied everyday life in West Papua. Nothing, it seems, is ever simple, patience is truly a virtue, and in the highlands, death a regular companion. In November Jessie updated her supporters on the catastrophic situation she had returned to.

Drought, death and desperation

I am back in Korupun! As I look back over the past few weeks of shifting scenes, cultures and priorities, my mind boggles. We seem to go from one drama to another....I spent a few days in Sentani getting all my paperwork organised. It was hot and the smog (from bushfires) was bad there too. I was able to get a seat on a MAF plane which was able to sneak through the drifting layers of smoke into Wamena. I stayed with Sue for four days until the smog lifted enough to get me home. Each day I would go to the MAF hangar and sit and wait for several hours and then go back to Sue's for another night. The sun was a bright red blob behind the heavy smoke layer. Then one morning it rained a little and cleared the air enough to take off.

The people were very pleased to see me back. They are planning a welcome back feast this week when all the clinic workers will be in for the event. When I stepped off the plane there was the sound of wailing. Someone had just died. In the past five months a mysterious illness has been raging amongst the Yali and Kimyal people. People often die within 12 to 24 hours of getting sick. There have been over 100 deaths in the past three months among the Kimyal people. Lots more in the Yali area.

Without any laboratory facilities it was a big jigsaw puzzle to try to fit together, mostly guess work and trial and error. At first it was thought to be Japanese encephalitis, then after a team of doctors came in it was thought to be bacterial meningitis, then after further tests it was proven to be cerebral malaria. We have never had the mosquito here so the people have really reacted badly to it. After months of very little food because of the drought their resistance is very low to this new malady. Usually these mosquitos won't survive at this altitude in the cold and wet weather. But this year, because of the long dry season and the lack of rain causing many streams to dry up and become stagnant pools, it is just right for them to breed. They are multiplying fast.

The wind and the sun continue to dry out the soil and it has made the people's gardens so hard they cannot dig them and the potatoes cannot grow. The future looks grim. I have been making big pots of soup to give out to those who cannot eat. This encourages them to drink.

I have been thankful for all the clinic workers who have taken on a lot of the workload and have delegated one village to each of the workers. They go each morning and evening to check on everyone, give injections as needed, and their medication. They also encourage them to drink. So many die simply because they stop drinking when they get sick. Then later on the 'soup lady' (me) goes around with a pot of soup and ladles it out at each house where there are sick people. In between all this we are busy at the clinic with the sick ones who can walk.

Attending funerals is not my favourite occupation but these past weeks have served as a reminder that death could strike at any time and we need to be ready to meet the Lord. It has been hard not being able to cure the sick because we are unsure of the cause. We are so thankful to have the bug identified and although we are very busy we are seeing positive results from our treatment.

We are thankful that the government and the Freeport Mining Company have been distributing some food by helicopter. Not nearly enough as there are thousands needing food. It has been very hard for them. Even the possums and the birds in the forests are dying of thirst. We are thankful that so far people still have clean drinking water. Many springs have dried up and others are just a trickle but still flowing. Of the 38 waterfalls around the valley only two continue to flow. I have been buying food for the people from some gifts that have been given for relief work. They are very grateful for anything that we can do for them. WE WOULD BE GLAD OF HELP FOR THIS PROJECT.

Even the little things in life were harder in the drought, the worst on record in the highlands of New Guinea.

Our hydro is not working, so I am back to using my old pressure lamp in the evenings. I am thankful for a good light. (November 1997)

Her sister Vera added some notes of her own to the letter:

'Jess does not mention such things as no power for electric jug, toaster, iron, fridge, deep freeze. All water, except what she is conserving for cooking and drinking has to be carted from the river. No hot showers now.'

Vera also included some information from a private letter to family.

Because we don't have any electricity I cannot use my word processor and have had to drag out my old typewriter that is over 30 years old....I should have gone out today to conference but the smoke was so bad in Wamena the plane couldn't take off. So I am working here tonight. I have a candle perched up on a box so I can see. Carol and Art Clark have been in the middle of all this sickness. They have had more people die than we have, about 74 altogether at Lolat. There are all sorts of medical teams coming in now. Sela has also been very bad.

Jessie's January 1998 prayer letter had a markedly different, exuberant tone:

The sound of steady pounding rain on the roof filled our hearts with thanksgiving for answered prayer. It has ended the drought, but not the famine. It will take six to nine months before the potatoes are ready to dig. One of the pilots said that he hadn't realised how badly the drought had affected him until it started to rain. The sound made him want to sing, dance and shout 'hallelujah' and run around in the rain. What a release to know the disaster is over.

We are thankful the cerebral malaria is under control and the Lord has sent rain to this thirsty land. The streams are flowing again and the waterfalls roaring. Wonderfully answered prayer from so many people worldwide. It has been exciting to see the change of attitude in the people who now see that they have HOPE for the future. Every able-bodied person is out making new gardens.

We praise the Lord for each one of you who has so generously given gifts to help buy extra food for the people. It has been a tremendous help and encouragement for us all. We have had offers of help from other aid organisations but they have been hampered by red tape and have not been able to get things moving as fast as they had hoped. With your gifts we have been able to quickly help where the need is most urgent. Thank you.

We started a feeding program for children under five years which has been greatly appreciated by the parents. We make a bean and rice porridge for them plus a cup of milk each morning. It is very popular. The children don't own such luxuries as cups, bowls and spoons. These had to be sent in from Wamena before the children's feeding program could commence. In between flights (which can be from four to seven days) the people have been living mainly on potato leaves and anything else they can find in the forest. They have been glad of the oil that has come in with the rice to make it more nourishing and palatable. A few weeks ago the children discovered mushrooms in the burnt out forest area. What a lovely surprise to add to their diet.

Some of the churches in other areas here in Irian that are not affected by the drought have sent potatoes, peanuts and corn. Our church gave bags of corn seed which was divided out between the drought-stricken areas. The people are really keen to plant anything that will make a quick harvest. MAF is really hard pressed to keep up flights with supplies to the affected areas. They asked for help from the Australian MAF in Papua New Guinea, They sent over two pilots with the Twin Otter for two weeks to help shift rice. It made sure everyone had rice for Christmas. We had to upgrade our airstrip by doing a lot of work on it to allow the wider wing span plane to land safely. You can imagine the mounting excitement when it actually landed. Most of the people have never seen a twin-engine plane before. It could shift 1800 kilos in one load whereas the Cessna can only shift 400 kilos.

The Christmas celebrations were a little different this year. Instead of eating the usual sweet potato, pork and vegies at the feasts, it was eating rice off a banana leaf with very little else. But it was a good time for fellowship.

The past week we have all come down with a bump as a new strain of flu has hit the valley. So many are sick. Because of their weakened condition they are not bouncing back as usual. Pneumonia and chest complaints have plagued the babies and older folk. The in-between age groups have had vomiting and diarrhoea with flu symptoms. I succumbed to it, and it knocked me flat for three days. I'm not sure what age bracket I should be in???

It takes a long time to recover from a drought of such gravity but people are resilient. Another 21 months passed before Jessie could report:

Yesterday an excited man came to tell me to praise the Lord that the pandanus nut trees are loaded with fruit. They should have a bumper crop this year. Many trees died or were burnt during the drought. This will be the first good crop since then. It will be a great blessing to everyone as they are short of potatoes and the nuts are rich in protein and oil.

25. Jessie's two worlds

I did not drive in Sydney. I chickened out and caught the train. Much safer for everyone.

The missionaries helped bring the outside world to remote parts of West Papua changing forever the world of the Indigenous population caught at the interface between cultures and beliefs. Yet the missionaries were also crossing a cultural divide, particularly long-term placements like Jessie. They lived in remote villages close to the people they were there to serve.

They had their own small, but tightly knit expatriate community which they relied heavily on for mutual support, particularly in time of crisis, ill-health and other personal difficulties. Most had home countries that they returned to during year-long furloughs that fell due every four years. Jessie was a Melbourne girl, and that became her base during the extended stays home in Australia. West Papua was modernizing at a steady but gradually increasing rate, from stone-age to a more modern society with a growing Christian community and the steady introduction of both Indonesian and western customs and concepts. Australia too was changing from the insular, inward looking, overwhelmingly Christian, Anglo-Saxon country Jessie left in 1966, to the modern, vibrant, increasingly confident, secular and multicultural society it is today. Jessie worked hard to maintain her Australian links with family, friends and supporters, traveling extensively and sharing her experiences whenever she returned to the country.

Time is flying fast as I get back into the swing of living here in Australia again. I have had the use of the mission car which has been a great help in getting round to visit people and also to take meetings. The little yellow 'colt' and I are getting broken in together. After four years of not driving it isn't easy to get back into the hurly burly of traffic again. When I got home it was suggested that it would be a good idea for me to join the ambulance fund! I'll let you decide on the reason why.

After a very busy time of deputations in Victoria I am now in central New South Wales. I have been so thankful for caring friends who offered to drive me north of Parkes to Nyngen, Bourke, Wee Waa, Gunnedah and Dubbo as they are long hours on the road with only the kangaroos and emus for company. I have just spent time in Sydney but was not brave enough to drive through it. I decided to leave the car at Katoomba and go by train. I set aside a day so that I could be at my niece's wedding which was a special day as I usually miss out on most of the family special times because I am too far away. I would value your prayer as I continue to travel around the Sydney area and then fly onto Queensland in July and back to Tasmania in August. I am planning to have some time off in September before flying back to Irian Jaya. (June 1992)

It is 30 years since I had a Christmas in Melbourne so it is special for me. Just six weeks before I left (West Papua) I was out taking the dog for a walk one evening when I slipped and fell. I guessed I had fractured my wrist. Of course it was too late to contact anyone that night so I bandaged it up and waited until morning to contact the mission doctor. He suggested an x-ray but first I had to get a plane to fly the one-and-a-half hours to get to Senggo Hospital. After the x-ray the doctor put me in plaster and I had to wait four days before I could get back to Korupun. (December 1996)

While homecomings were always eagerly anticipated they didn't always bring the rest and recreation Jessie expected.

The saga all started when I returned home and some of my friends spoilt me by making some very special meals with lots of cream cheese in them. My poor old gall bladder wasn't used to coping with such rich food and re-belled by giving me some uncomfortable nights. Then to add insult to injury one of the gall stones decided he wanted to move house and got stuck in the bile duct. This caused great concern and pain until it moved on and lodged somewhere else. Medical advice was that if it happened again whilst I was in Irian Jaya it would be quite dangerous, so I am happy to leave them behind me. It was quite a different experience to be on the other side of the sheets for a change. I was pleasantly surprised to find it wasn't as bad as expected. The new 'keyhole' surgery certainly makes convalescence much quicker as they don't cut through any muscles. I was out in two days. At the moment I am still recuperating and have been thankful for all the good nurses and the open homes to help me convalesce.

It is always hard to get back into the traffic again after not driving for four years. Lots of new road rules and highways to get me confused. I have finally learnt how to negotiate the new ring road without causing a major traffic jam. (June 1997)

Jessie prudently planned for eventual retirement back in Melbourne and as the years crept by, that planning was bearing fruit.

Some of you have been asking about the status of my unit for my retirement. I have had tenants in it helping to pay off the mortgage and I do praise the Lord that it is now paid off. I will need some alterations, new carpets, etc. before I move in, but I am not exactly sure when that will be. (June 1997)

Vera had long been the conduit between Jessie and her Australian network, retyping hundreds of her sister's prayer letters and other news from West Papua, and mailing them out on Jessie's behalf. Later that year Vera shared more information on Jessie's retirement plans.

'A big decision for us as well as Jessie. Ken and I have decided to have our home demolished and have two units built on the block – one for us and one for Jessie. Both homes needed to be updated and this way we will both end up with homes that hopefully 'will see us out!' Plans for both units are with the local council waiting for approval to build. Jessie will sell her existing unit to finance her new unit. Many of you have spoken of contributing to her unit when she retires. Now is the time to do it as extras cost money – i.e. curtains, carpets, light fittings. Another sister, Jean Dundas, is overseeing the building of Jessie's unit. If you would like to contribute please send gifts to Jean but made payable to 'Jessie Williamson' so that they can go directly to Jessie's account.'

The transition to retirement always takes some adjustment - much more so when the two worlds you inhabit are so wide apart.

This year will also hold a lot of changes for me as I will be retiring from Irian at the end of the year. I will probably be working in the mission office a few days a week, as well as doing deputations when I get home. Do pray that I will make this year count for His glory and that everything that has been planned will get done. Pray too that I will be mentally and physically prepared for the transition. (March 2000)

Sue and I are praising the Lord that our new visas have been granted for another year. I was particularly glad to receive mine so that I could come home for my annual medical and also to see my sister Vera who has just recently been diagnosed with leukemia. She has just had one course of chemo and is due for another next month. She is in remission at present. (June 2000)

While Vera battled leukemia, Jessie moved towards inevitable retirement from the field.

I would value your prayer as I start to clear out 30+ years of stuff I have accumulated, wither to send it, lend it or give it to whoever has the biggest need. It all takes time. I guess I will have a big bonfire in the end. I hope to be home in January. Do pray for me in these last few months that I will be able to do all that I have planned. Pray for all the different ones who will be taking over new responsibilities in the next three months as we plan to close the station. I will need your prayers in a new life as I try to settle into life at home in Melbourne. It is always a traumatic experience to get back into a car and into traffic plus learning my way round the new freeways and highways. Thank you so much for your support over the past 35 years. I will continue to need your support for a couple more years yet as I plan to be working part time in the Mission Office. (September 2000)

26. Earthquakes

I woke at 12.15 am (19 January 1981) to find my bed rocking violently, the house shaking, cracking and moaning.

Geologists now believe the earth's crust is comprised of a series of about 40 mostly large plates that crush against each other with incredible force. The northern edge of the Australian Plate runs from Cocos Islands in the Indian Ocean in the west to New Caledonia in the Pacific Ocean to the east where it turns south towards New Zealand. The route of this seismic belt is commonly referred to as the 'Pacific Rim of Fire'. It is one of the most seismically active zones on earth, experiencing a third of all recorded earthquakes on our planet. The 'Rim of Fire' virtually dissects the island of New Guinea from west to east. Somewhere close to Korupun the northern rim of the Australian Plate presses flush against the mighty Pacific Plate, the largest of the crust plates covering a touch more than 20 per cent of the earth's surface. Over eons of time the pressure of these plates pushing against each other created the mighty mountain chain that runs along the spine of the island of New Guinea.

Jessie probably gave no thought to the powerful forces shifting beneath her when she bedded down on the night of Sunday 18 January. To that point the forces moving deep within the earth's surface would have been imperceptible even though, in geological terms, the Australian Plate was pushing north-north-east at a breakneck speed of six to seven centimetres a year. The pressure was building and something was about to give. At 15 minutes after midnight a large earthquake registering 6.8 on the Richter scale shook Jessie's mountain domain.

Before I was properly awake I was out of bed and headed toward the back door. It was like trying to walk on board a ship in a gale. Things falling off the shelves, with plates and cups tumbling out of cupboards made my progress an obstacle race. Such a mess to clean up later. As I tried to open the door I was flung against it, banging my nose and spraining my wrist. At last I was outside the house and wondering if the house would hold together. Shivering in my pyjamas with bare feet and the rain pouring down, made life rather uncomfortable. After what seemed a long time to me, in reality a few minutes, it settled down somewhat, and I ventured inside to get a torch, coat and gumboots to go down and see how Elinor had fared. She had polio as a child and is a little unsteady on her feet. She stayed in bed. We turned on the radio to see if anyone else had been affected. Lolat (Seng Valley) and Holowon both came on to say they were shaken but OK. The centre of the earthquake was between Lolat and Korupun in the Solo Valley. So our two stations were the most shook up. Others barely felt it.

We continued to have tremors and aftershocks about every 15 minutes all night so we didn't get a great deal of sleep. Just as I was dozing off about 4 am there was a terrific roar from the mountain near my home. Then the sound of tearing and rending as part of the side of the mountain gave way in a large landslide. It hit the river with a tremendous thud, sending dust and spray billowing 200 feet into the air. The next morning we looked around the valley and there were about 10 landslides. One has come perilously near the village. Two women were reported missing but were later found.

The earthquake's epicentre was in Yali country between the valleys of the Seng River to the west and its tributary the Solo River to the east. This placed the epicentre some 25-40 kilometres west of Korupun. Where Korupun was badly shaken the Solo Valley was devastated. Official figures put the death toll at about 300, though it may well have been higher.

Thousands of others were hurt, lost their homes and crops and many were forced off their land.

Although it was bad here, it is nothing to the devastation in the Solo Valley. They say the whole valley is denuded of vegetation and looks very like the Grand Canyon. Ten villages were either swept away or destroyed and most of the people from all of these villages have disappeared under the landslides. A few people have been miraculously saved and the helicopter has picked them up and placed them all together. Thus in a valley of approximately 2000 population there are now very few. In the next valley from us one house and family were swept away by the landslide. The father managed amazingly to escape. The next morning as they were viewing the scene of the disaster they suddenly heard a child crying. Investigating, they discovered the child still alive under the landslide and they were able to dig her out. They said she was curled up like a little worm in the earth with no injuries except fright. In another incident a boy was buried up to his neck and was safely dug out the next morning. Ones and twos here and there but the majority suddenly swept into eternity.

Two of our villages closer to the Solo Valley were badly affected and a runner came in next day with news that the people were stranded between landslides with no food. Their gardens had been swept away, the landslide is still moving and it is unsafe to travel. They were hungry. Elinor and I went by MAF helicopter to take them food and to check the injured. We took rice, potatoes, vitamins, soup and pots to cook in.... One lady had been killed by a falling rock and another badly injured after her house collapsed on her. We brought her back with us in the helicopter. (January 1981)

Les Henson also has vivid memories of the earthquake and its aftermath:

'The sides of the Seng Valley, I think south of Lolat, collapsed with landslides and formed a large lake, which burst open about two to three weeks after the initial earthquake and sent a mini tsunami into the lowlands. The Akin River on which we were located at Sumo rose 20 feet inside one hour.'

It was a difficult time in the quake zone with the missions, as always, playing a central role in relief efforts. Jessie kept her network informed on progress.

My sincere thanks to those of you who were able to help us with our earthquake needs....We hope to slowly start phasing out the rice supplement after the next six weeks. Their gardens should be producing sufficient then. We have had a very long dry season this year and that has been very helpful for those needing to build new homes and gardens. (May 1981)

Earthquakes were an unfortunate fact of life in West Papua. On 1 August 1989, at 9.17 am local time, another earthquake – this one registering 6.0 on the Richter scale – struck in Dani and Yali areas in the Lower Grand Valley west of Korupun. This quake also caused serious landslides and flooding which claimed 120 lives. All of the dead were recovered from the villages of Holowon, Pasema and Soba where Jessie's friend Sue Trenier lived.

Last month we had an earthquake and its centre was at Soba which is 30 air-miles from here. We were all down at the airstrip saying goodbye to some visitors when the ground started to heave and rock under our feet. The plane started to sway and the pilot thought it was a pig in the pod jumping around until he saw his passenger absolutely terrified covering their heads with their arms. We had no real damage here but the Soba area was devastated. Sue was in her office when it struck. She said it felt like a giant hand had hit the side of the house knocking them off their feet and sprawling across the room. Books and papers were flying around and Sue lost her glasses in the melee. They all rushed out to the airstrip for safety. The other mission house fell down and Sue's was leaning at a 45 degree angle. Then one by one the landslides started to rumble and gather momentum on all sides. The mountains were quickly divested of all vegetation, people, gardens and houses. The debris from the landslides blocked up the big Baliem River and dammed back the water making a big lake. This was a concern in case it broke and took more villages with it.

The MAF helicopter happened to be in the area and the plane that had taken off from here was there in 10 minutes. As soon as he got back to

Wamena David (the pilot) jumped out of his plane into the other helicopter and took off. He had picked up John Wilson to act as eyes and MAF swung into action as a search and rescue operation as soon as the dust settled from the initial landslides. John said the pilots were fantastic as they hovered over with just one skid on a rock on the steep mountains. They had to be careful not to hit the mountain with the rotor blades. John would then jump out and check the people, and if alive, help them into the helicopter. The people they found stranded or injured were then taken to Sue for assessment and either taken to hospital or taken to a safer village which had not been affected.

Because of the big mudslide at the back of Sue's house and the fact the ground was unstable there with six big cracks in the airstrip, Sue was evacuated to Owakbasik with the 1000 refugees they had collected from around the valley. It was the first time in months that both the helicopters had been ready for use. (They were always waiting for parts). Now begins the long task of keeping people fed until they can plant gardens. The government is very keen for them to be relocated but the people are not happy to move. This is inherited land. Do pray for all the decisions that have to be made.

This past week I have been running off 200 copies of I and II Corinthians in the Soba language (40 stencils) on the duplicator for Sue to distribute at Owakbasik and the other refugee village. She just finished translating this before the quake and of course now has no way of getting it done. She thought that whilst the people had time on their hands they could practice their reading. Where the people have heard about the disaster at Soba they want to help their fellow believers. Although they don't have a great deal themselves they all brought potatoes enough to fill a plane to send to the Soba people. Out of their little they gave much. (September 1989)

Not surprisingly most of Jessie's private letters to family around this time mentioned the earthquake.

August 10: Today they had another small quake which has caused more mud and landslides to come down. Now several other villages are threatened and they have to decide what to do with 800 more refugees. They are at 7000 feet so it is very cold. I sent over lots of little knitted singlets that many of you have made for the children. It should make a splash of colour and also keep the children warm. The people are going out to salvage pieces of houses wrecked by the landslides to make new homes. There is a shortage of housing with the influx of all those people. With most of the gardens gone it is hard for them. Sue is living in the village with the people and organising the distribution of the food the government sends in. She said for days the people were in shock, very dazed and had to be forced to eat. Almost everyone there has lost someone, and many, everyone. They are all grieving for loved ones swept away.

September 1: Very hard on the helicopter pilots and one nearly crashed when he got caught in a sudden change of cloud formation. They are delivering rice to the earthquake people every other day. The government is pushing for villagers to relocate but it is hard for them to make a decision when they are still in a state of shock. Sue is still living up there with the 900 refugees. Following the earthquake, many people around Soba were homeless so the government saw this as an opportunity to relocate them nearer the town. For those people who had never been on a plane it was exciting but gradually they just walked nine or 10 days back again.

Almost a year later villagers were still struggling to rebuild their lives and livelihoods. Following the dedication of a new church and the graduation service for Bible school students Jessie reported:

I was given a pregnant mother pig as a thank you offering for having trained the clinic worker for them. I decided I didn't really need a pig so I have since sent it off to Soba to help the people there get their pig breeding started again. They lost nearly all their pigs in the earthquake. (June 1990)

27. An inspiration to many

The Lord has sent along quite a number of visitors lately which has been wonderful to break the loneliness for me. (June 2000)

'Jessie has the gift of hospitality. She is always ready to give a cup of tea with cookies/biscuits and a meal or a bed for those who stop by accidentally (due to weather or medical emergency) or on purpose. Jessie entertained, and often would have a houseful of guests. She always had a place and always served good meals in spite of her busy schedule.'

– Kathryn Kline.

Rosa Kidd has similar memories:

'When you minister in a small station together there is naturally a lot of interaction. Orin and I were the married couple and then besides us there were two single gals, Elinor and Jessie. We were partners in ministry but we were also friends. Aside from our Kimyal friends, we were each other's only social contact for months at a time. We invited each other over for meals, went on picnics and treks together and almost always had our Sunday meal and evening service together. We even had ladies nights when Orin was banned and we just had some female bonding time. Every morning at 10 am and then again at 3 pm Jessie, Elinor, Orin and I would rotate to one another's houses for our morning and afternoon coffee breaks. This was a time for sharing what was going on in our separate ministries, a time to pray with one another and to share our home and family news. It gave us all a break from the stresses of our work. An extra blessing of those coffee breaks is that Jessie always shared with us some of her special goodies that she received from her friends and family back in Australia.'

For Sue Trenier, Christmas at Korupun was a special time:

'I often went to Korupun to spend Christmas, staying with Jessie and enjoying the break and fellowship with the missionary team there. However she managed it I don't know but we always had endless presents to open, lots of meals and feasts with the locals, lovely music to listen to and endless 'cuppas' over which we chewed the rag for hours. We shared and chatted and also took walks around the area where Jessie was well loved and accepted.'

Other times they took a Christmas break together visiting other mission communities, as usual, sharing the novel experiences with those back home.

Sue and I ended up going to the south coast for Christmas to be with the Mills family. It was very hot and sultry and of course the lowland people are very different from the highlanders. It was interesting to be part of a different kind of Christmas celebration. No pig feasts like we were used to having. Instead we had sago grubs (like witcherty grubs) and perpeda which is made from sago. Of course everyone watched with great interest to see how we would cope. We decided the grubs were tough and tasteless but we kept them down. The perpeda is made by pouring hot water on the sago flour and stirring it until it is a glutinous mess like old fashioned starch clag, and they love it. The local people all cooked their own food in their own square houses and brought it to the airstrip to eat. They all sat on their own woven mats. (February 1993)

But Jessie's hospitality and conviviality wasn't restricted to close friends as Sue recalls:

'I have an Indonesian doctor friend who worked for a time in Karabuga where he heard many good things about 'Yetty' and was keen to meet her. Some years later he made a visit to Korupun. At that time Jessie was the only expat in Korupun. Dr Andreas was no doubt used to the various conditions he could meet on a medical visit to interior areas. When he arrived in Korupun though he was directed to a guest house with a guest room all prepared – bed, sheets, towels etc. – and on the table a vase with a bunch of roses and a note welcoming him and hoping his stay and ministry in Korupun would be a blessing and that he would be a blessing to the Kimyals. He was very moved, especially when he found special foodstuffs in the kitchen and so forth. He was truly blessed by Jessie's thoughtfulness and practical love shown him and it remains with him to this day.'

Hospitality was just one of the many qualities that endeared Jessie to people.

'Jessie is a very good encourager, remembering folks with birthday cards, especially to all the children in the mission. Jessie is a gift giver as well. Her supporters gave her little gifts and cards for her 'Encouraging' ministry. She will be remembered by a good number of people for this gift. Jessie is also a prayer warrior. This goes along with her correspondence ministry of informing folks of news and prayer requests to her constituents of how and what to pray.' – Kathryn Kline.

'Jessie impacted many lives for Christ during her years of service in West Papua, both among the tribal people as well as the missionary community – many missionary children were delivered by Jessie.' – Rosa Kidd.

Since I last wrote to you I have been helping at the small Team Hospital on the South Coast. While there, two missionaries had babies and the plane on which I was scheduled to leave arrived with an emergency caesarean section. The pilot decided to stay overnight as it was late in the afternoon, so I hastily donned theatre attire to 'scrub' for the operation. A healthy 5lb boy was the result. (August 1967)

'On various occasions she spent holiday time with us at Holowon, which gave the opportunity for her to get to know our family, and for our three boys to come to know her as Auntie Jessie – as she became for all the missionary kids in Irian Jaya. And for decades afterwards, without fail, they would receive a card or an email on their birthdays.' – John and Gloria Wilson.

'For me personally Jessie was family, somehow she always made her family my family which encouraged me to do the same. She has a great understanding of Christians as family, not least how she sent birthday cards to missionary kids for years and also many, many people like myself to whom she never forgets to send a birthday card.'

– Sue Trenier

Being a midwife meant Jessie often spent time with other missionary families during late pregnancy and at child birth, a special time in every family's life, made even more so by the peculiar circumstances of missionary life so far away from their closest family and friends.

When a missionary is due to have her baby the whole family is flown in here three weeks before the due date. The family does all the cooking so that relieves me of the responsibility. (August 1966)

MAF called to say they had on board a missionary lady who went into labour five weeks prematurely. Organised another plane to borrow a humi-crib from the Mulia Hospital which arrived just in time for a little 4lb 8oz baby girl. All well. (July 1975)

This past month I have also helped in some medical emergencies among our own missionaries. I was asked to go to Mulia to help look after Janet and Dale Brown's little premature baby. It seems it was baby month as Kathryn Kline began to have complications in her delivery and needed to go to Papua New Guinea for a caesarean section. I was asked to go along in case there were any complications en-route. The only one we encountered was the fact that it was Independence Day in PNG and a holiday so the officials were not too pleased at having to come to clear us through customs, immigration, etc. Someone jokingly said 'here comes the flying nurse again'. (October 1978).

She gave more detail of baby Brown's birth in a letter to family.

At the moment I am trying to prop my eyelids open as I am sitting watching a little three pound nine ounce premature baby. The Browns who have been here only a couple of months had a six weeks premature baby yesterday much to everyone's shock. As he needs constant care at the moment they asked if I could come and help with the round the clock care. So here I am at Mulia once again. It is in the highlands so it is cool. They had the baby in the humi-crib yesterday but the generator broke down so now we are managing with hot water bottles. So far he is doing just fine so we are praying he will continue to do so. (August 1978)

Jess regularly reported back on visitors to Korupun.

We recently had a work team from the USA here to build two new classrooms for the Bible School. It was great to see it go ahead so quickly in the two weeks. They got the foundations, frame, roof and floor in before the wood ran out. The local carpenters are putting on the siding as it comes to hand. (May 1995)

I got back to Korupun just in time to welcome a group of men from the USA. Dr David Gee was here last year and this time he brought two of his friends with him. Chris was a builder who was able to help Sabil build an office cum guest house. (August 1995)

One of Jessie's many visitors was Reverend Geoff Shepherd, now chaplain to the Richmond Football Club and senior pastor at the Mill Park Baptist Church in Melbourne. In an interview published on the Baptist Union of Victoria website he was asked: 'Who do you admire?' He listed his parents and a small number of others.

'I've got a few heroes, mainly unsung ones,' Geoff replied. 'I admire Jessie Williamson, who I first met in Korupun, Irian Jaya. This humble nurse served 'til she retired in the Irianese highlands under conditions which would send most of us running away today.'

Geoff was not the only young person to find inspiration in the humble, and humbling, circumstances of Korupun. Rosa Orin recounts 'Nellie's story':

'Nellie was a young university student who came out with our summer short term program. She came out looking for excitement and wanting to visit a remote and exotic part of the world. Shortly after Nellie's arrival it was reported that there were two medical emergencies in one of our outlying areas. The first was a very young girl who was having trouble delivering a baby, and the second a seriously ill patient that needed to be seen by a doctor. We arranged for a helicopter to pick them up and bring them first to Korupun, so they could be evaluated by Jessie to determine whether they could be cared for at Korupun, or would need to be sent on to Wamena where there was a hospital. The helicopter landed and Jessie had to make a quick assessment and decision regarding both patients. Being a midwife she felt she could help the girl in labour but sent the other patient on to Wamena. What they didn't tell her in those hurried minutes at the airstrip was that the young girl had been in labour already for four days. After the helicopter left, Jessie, myself and Nellie took the patient and got her settled so Jessie could take a better look at her. What she found was that labour had stopped the day before and the baby was stuck in the birth canal. Jessie started her on medication to restart labour while I worked to calm the patient and her anxious husband who was very fearful that she was going to die.

Unfortunately, the girl was too small to deliver the baby and Jessie decided to do an episiotomy. So here is the picture! Jessie, Nellie, the patient and I are in one of the small, dark Kimyal huts. The girl is fearful and crying while I am by her head trying to calm her and explain what Jessie is going to do to help her deliver her baby. Nellie is holding the flashlight on the girl while Jessie does the episiotomy and delivers the baby. Jessie finally gets the baby out but it is not breathing. She needs to attend to the girl because she is losing lots of blood and needs to be sewn up. So, since Nellie is close to the baby,

Jessie gives her a hypodermic needle and tells her to poke the baby in the bottom to stimulate it to cry and breath. Nellie starts saying that she can't do it but realizes that this is life or death for both baby and mother. She finds herself doing something she would never have imagined and that was totally out of the realm of her expectations for this trip.

Even though many prayers were going up to heaven the baby did not survive. The mother did but had severe nerve damage from the extended pressure of the baby on her groin and was paralysed and unable to walk. Jessie gave Nellie the job of caring for this 14-year old girl, which she did with much compassion and tenderness for the next three weeks she was with us. That summer we had several obstructed labour patients and other very sick people in the village right around us. One was a middle of the night call to help a woman with a retained placenta. Nellie and I went as interpreter and assistant. Having these very personal encounters with the Kimyal people had a life changing impact. At the end of summer Nellie was sharing her thoughts about what she had learned through her experiences. She mentioned that she had come to Korupun for excitement, but He had given her a calling! Nellie returned home to take training as a nurse and give her life to helping others.'

Jessie also enjoyed playing host to the infrequent but welcome visits from her family.

This past week I went out to Sentani to meet my sister Thelma and her husband Jim. Jim is a dentist so had promised that he would teach the clinic workers how to pull teeth the right way. They were all keen and listened well and seemed to catch on to the procedures. The proof of the pudding is in the eating and I guess it will be the end results that will tell. Jim pulled several teeth and he had them all clustered around wanting to see it all. Pray for them and that I will be able to get them some old dental forceps to use. I also had several sessions with them upgrading and teaching them new concepts etc. It was a busy four days. (March 1994)

This past month my sister Jean and niece Judy were here for four weeks – an unexpected pleasure. During that time I had planned to go to Sumo, in the southern lowlands to give a refresher course to the clinic workers there. (So they came along too). The lowland people are not as energetic as the highland tribes (due largely to the humid climate and incessant malaria). However 15 of them turned up for the course. (May 1995)

My nephew Paul had quite a few different experiences whilst he was here. I had to attend an Eastern Highlands Clinic Workers Conference at Soba for part of that time, so he tagged along. Some 70 people attended including the head of the health department for Irian Jaya, head of the health department for our area and clinic workers from the four different tribes in the Eastern Highlands. Each delegate had to bring food to help with the menu. We had quite a few delicacies such as fried rice with turtle meat, several sago dishes, dried deer meat and noodles, roast pork and pork cooked in the pit etc. We ran out of eggs so I used turtle eggs to bake biscuits and cake for morning tea and they were quite tasty. (February 1996)

28. Rebels, war and payback

Before Christmas everything seemed quiet, but then right after Christmas there was a rebel flare up about a day's walk from here, ending in the massacre of 75 people including women and children. Some Karubaga folk were killed.

With the coming of Christianity, western ideas, Indonesian colonisation and new examples of material wealth, expectations naturally rose among the local Papuan peoples. By 1974 Jessie had been long enough in the highlands to appreciate the impact the arrival of these foreign cultures and concepts could have. She was also aware that western concepts of education and opportunity brought with them expectations and that these expectations could not always be met.

Do continue to pray for our young people that they will not be dissatisfied after they have struggled through six grades of school to suddenly find themselves at a loose end as there are only a few openings for further education. Youth with nothing to occupy its restlessness finds mischief to get into and our young people are no exception. (August 1974)

They were prescient comments. For it was not only the young that felt alienated in their own lands. Nor was it only the arrival of missionaries that disrupted the balance of traditional Papuan life, for the missions also felt threatened by the encroachment of Indonesian authority across Papuan territory. A fledgling Papuan nationalist movement emerged in the immediate aftermath of Indonesia's takeover from the Dutch. Discontentment simmered as Nationals found themselves locked out of many of the better paid official government jobs. When they looked longingly across the border to Papua New Guinea which gained full independence from Australia in 1975 the Indonesian yoke grated even more harshly. Jessie shared some of their concerns.

Next year, 1977, may see changes here as Indonesia will again be plunged into elections. The Muslim party is desperately trying to gain control and if they do, it may mean the end of evangelical missions and freedom of religion in Indonesia.

As the election approached, tensions rose.

Do pray for Indonesia in the days ahead as the elections loom closer to us. It is a time of much unrest and tension. We will all need the love and wisdom from the Lord to cope with the many new demands that will be made upon us. (April 1977)

The rebel movement, known as the Organisasi Papua Merdeka (OPM) or Papuan Independence Organisation, asserted itself, raised its profile and began a vigorous recruitment drive. There was a groundswell of local support, particularly among the disaffected young. Les Henson provides the background:

'The rebels were largely made up of people from the north coast of West Papua and many Danis mainly from the Australian Pacific Christian Mission (APCM) and the Christian and Missionary Alliance (C&MA) areas of work and ministry. During late 1976 and 1977 there was incredible turmoil throughout the greater Dani region as the OPM began to recruit people to their cause. Those who stood against the movement were often killed and mutilated. By the end of 1977 the movement was dying out in the Dani region. Many of the missionary leaders and church leaders spoke against the movement because of the false hope of independence from the Indonesian government and forces, it presented.'

Jessie informed both her family and prayer network of the troubles, though she seemed to understate, rather than overstate the risks and dangers involved.

I guess you have heard about some of our troubles up here. (Fighting between the tribes). We were all evacuated by helicopter three weeks ago but have since been able to return. Most of the unrest and tension has settled in our area although other areas are still unsettled. (May 1977)

Things have settled down here again and we hope for a while but one never knows. We haven't been in any danger from the people but were evacuated because they thought we might get caught between the two opposing parties. (June 1977)

She was clearly struggling to make sense of the complex situation, a potent cocktail of politics, religion, power structures and ambitions.

We are back into the swing of everyday work. Do pray for other areas that are not back to normal and where there is much turmoil and strife. Many unbelievers and some weak believers have gone back to fetish making and spirit appeasement. The heathen have used this situation to get their own back on the Christians and have caused much heartbreak and loss. I will continue to supervise and work in the baby and antenatal clinics. Do pray for wisdom in diagnosing and treating these little ones now that the children have come back after they all fled to the forest for those weeks of trouble. I will be starting the children's program again on Tuesday. (August 1977)

On 27 December 1977 Jessie was taking a break at Lake Holmes, a humid, hot, but not unbearable location. In a family letter she wrote;

We had been rejoicing that the rebels were about all gone when we heard that they had come back into the APCM Bokondini area and killed 16 Dani Christians because they wouldn't join their rebel activities.

On 23 January a further update.

When I returned from Lake Holmes everyone here was carrying weapons. After the massacre our folk started patrolling the trails just in case they came this way. All was quiet until New Year's Eve when the cry went up that they were close by. So John (presumably mission administrator John Dekker) *and I had to sleep at Winnie's house for the night. We celebrated the New Year waiting for an attack that never came. A boy has just come to the door to say they are off on the track of some more rebels four hours in the other direction. I am glad they can see where they are going. I would be sure to fall off a cliff at this time of night.*

In her February prayer letter Jessie gave a fuller account of the Bokondini massacre where 75 people died. Presumably the 16 Dani Christians mentioned in her earlier letter were among those killed.

This really roused the people into drastic action to rid the area of the rebels. Clan ties were forgotten as they realised the danger to their women and children. Some 500 warriors from here went to help the Bokondini people chase them out. A week later they returned home and created much excitement by performing a victory dance on the airstrip to let off steam and some of their feelings. We trust that this means the back of the rebel movement is broken in our area, although the people say there are still rebels hiding in the forests on the top of mountains. For this reason all of the people are still carrying their bows and arrows. Their weapons are never far from them as they work. There are still some areas that have not yet surrendered.

The last few Sundays the churches have been mainly filled with women, children and old men, while the younger men have stood guard outside in case of a surprise attack. But today the church came back to normal. There has been some talk in some areas of 'payback and revenge' by the non-Christians for those killed. I am also treating a lady who got mixed up with the rebel activity. She got a big gash in her thigh from an axe, a spear in her side (spear was deflected from her rib and amazingly caused no real damage) and about 10 arrow wounds in her back as she was running away. Her baby was grabbed off her back and killed as she fled.

Les Henson also recalls the massacre and its aftermath.

'The Bokondini massacre was one of the final events of the movement before the Indonesian government gained control of the area and many of its members became disillusioned and began to leave in droves. The remaining group of OPM members filtered down into the northern lowlands and into the Lake Plains area. But from that time the OPM was discredited among the Dani peoples. I remember being at Karubaga over the Christmas and New Year period building the penstock (main pipe) for the Hydro. The Dani men who worked with me carried their bows and arrows and had lookouts in case of attack from the Bokondini rebels.'

While Jessie often refers to the rebels she never mentions the OPM by name. Les Henson, knowing well the sensitivities of the times and the precarious position of the missions, surmises why:

'Part of the reason Jessie would not refer to the OPM would be that letters may have been monitored by the Indonesian Government. Thus she needed to be careful what she wrote and any reference to the OPM could not be direct. Also the OPM did not impact the Swart/ Toli valley to the same extent as other mission areas, because of the stand taken by RMBU's John Dekker and the local leaders against the movement.'

Les also recalls how Jessie responded to John Dekker's attempts to impose a night curfew during the period of heightened tensions in Karubaga. She simply ignored it on the basis that *no rebels going to dictate to me what I can and cannot do.*

Once the OPM issue settled, life returned to normal, but normal in the highlands could also have a dangerous edge, and the ever present threat of local justice, known as payback.

Yesterday I had just laid down after dinner for my siesta when Bill (MAF pilot) came to the door and said that one of the outposts had called and said that a fellow there had been hit with a bush knife and was bleeding to death. So I rushed around and grabbed my box of supplies plus a lot of extra bandages and we took off. As we landed there were people along the sides of the airstrip jumping up and down, all painted up, with their bow and arrows. They told us when we got there that if the man died there was going to be a full scale war and they were biding their time. He had two big slashes across his back and they were dripping blood. The teacher had tried to bandage him up but the relatives kept taking off the bandages!! So I bandaged him up and brought him with us on the plane and gave him a talking to about removing the bandage. Gave him a whopping dose of penicillin and trust it will heal. So one never knows what will happen next. (January 1979)

The West Papuan independence movement remained active. The mass transmigration of Indonesians from Java and other Indonesian islands which have little in common with the Melanesian Papuans aggravated local concerns, resulted in regular uprisings and outpourings of nationalist sentiment. The taking of five western hostages in 1996 again focused international attention on the plight of Papuans.

Of course, you have all heard about the hostage situation. It is situated about one hour flying from here and many miles to walk through jungle. We have not been affected but MAF and C&MA have been very involved. (February 1996)

Thank you for praying for the release of the hostages who have been held for the past five months. We were thrilled when it finally happened. We were saddened to hear that two of the National hostages had been killed by the rebels. We believe they were Christians. Two months before their release they had asked the Red Cross to get Bibles to all the captives. The folk at Wamena had supplied them with English, Dutch, German and Indonesian Bibles. (May 1996)

While the taking of European hostages made international headlines, Jessie's prayer letters also kept her network informed of the more routine business of tribal violence and payback.

Just before Christmas, we received news from Deibula that two men were presumed drowned after they failed to return from a hunting trip. Their dog came home without them. They searched for days along the river for their bodies and finally found them minus their heads. That put a very different complexion on the story. Foul play, but who was the culprit? Then a lady confessed that she had come across the place where they had been killed, but was too scared to tell anyone. They now know which village was responsible, but not who or why. The two villages involved have been busily employed in making bows and arrows. The hotheads in each place want to fight. The elders are trying to keep it under control. They do not want the payback system to start again – just the right people brought to justice. (March 1999)

Each year between Christmas and New Year the young people have a volleyball competition. In the Sela Valley one of the high school boys did not agree with the referee and punched him on the nose. Of course there was retaliation and before long all the spectators were involved. It then escalated to the whole village in the thick of it with bows and arrows, sticks and stones flying around. Some 60 people kept the clinic busy. The three main villages of Mondon, Gwarangdua and Megnum were caught up in the fighting and of course the non-believers had a field day. Now the elders and pastors are trying to sort it all out and repair the damage done between fragile relationships. (March 2000)

29. Rising expectations

The new millennium slipped in here at Korupun without any fanfare or fireworks. I wonder what this New Year will hold for our people of Irian Jaya. So many hopes and expectations are in the air.

As Jessie approached retirement she wrote more and more often about the rising tide of Papuan hopes for independence, with all the ambiguities and complexity it entailed. The main centre of Jayapura, and closer to home, Wamena, were at the heart of local agitation. From the relative calm and safety of Korupun, Jessie kept her network informed of developments with the growing Freedom Movement which was quite literally rallying around the Papuan flag, the powerful symbol of independence. Her potted history gives a real sense of the excitement, tensions and barely suppressed violence that were sweeping the highlands.

Special gatherings, rallies, marches plus the raising of the new flag have kept excitement and tensions high in the towns. Underneath the reasonably calm exterior things are bubbling and it could easily erupt given the right provocation. Pray for the leaders and the pastors as they endeavour to keep a tight rein on emotions that are riding high. The military have given a show of strength in the larger towns over the past months, especially in December when they put up the flag for a day. The pastors took the opportunity to preach to the crowds who were sitting around the flagpoles to explain what real freedom really means. It is freedom of the spirit towards God which does not rely on circumstances or flags. The government was impressed by the orderly way it was held. When they had a problem in another area they asked the pastors to go there and preach to the people. The next 'BIG' day was to be the 2nd of May but we have just heard it has been changed to December. (March 2000)

'Meredeka, Freedom, Meredeka, Freedom' was shouted from hundreds of throats as people converged on the city of Jayapura waving the new West Papuan Flag. They circled the city seven times and then sat peacefully outside the government offices. The expectations of the Freedom Movement plus the raising and lowering of the new flag so many times in the last three months has triggered off great excitement for independence. The church leaders have been trying to restrain the people from doing anything rash, but many will not listen to common sense any more. Praise the Lord that riots have thus far been avoided, mainly because the local people couldn't be bribed to start a ruckus. But thwarted hopes may boil over in the weeks and months ahead. In spite of all the marches and meetings etc. in the towns, life at Korupun has gone along quietly and steadily. (June 2000)

By now Jessie seemed more sympathetic to the independence movement then she was in earlier times though her biggest concern, as always, was to stop the violence.

The promised upheaval took place in Wamena three weeks ago when the people were told to take down all the new Papuan flags which had been proudly flying for several weeks. They refused to take them down, and when someone tried to do so, it was the spark that ignited the explosion. There was war on the streets of Wamena as people vented their frustration on people from other islands who were not Papuan. MAF quickly and smoothly moved into evacuation plans. All mission personnel were sent out to Sentani. MAF migrant workers were also flown out leaving a skeleton staff behind. At noon just when things were becoming very heated and MAF extra busy with 100 people wanting to be moved out a group of 20 tourists suddenly arrived at their door demanding to be evacuated immediately which added to the confusion. They were taken to a nearby airstrip out of the danger zone until they could be moved the next day. The Papuans went wild and chaos reigned. Houses were burnt, people killed and wounded and homes looted.

The helicopter was busy helping with the evacuees as well as shuffling the wounded from the other side of town across the fighting zone to the hospital. Unfortunately most of the doctors and hospital staff had fled except for two local doctors and clinic workers. The doctors were not surgeons. The Hercules air force planes were shuttling troops from Jayapura to Wamena. The situation continued to deteriorate later in the afternoon and it was thought wise to move the MAF planes to a safer location for the night. The helicopter stayed on the mission compound but was ready for a quick take-off with the four male missionaries who were left behind. The military were lenient and tried to only wound and not kill people, but if it comes to a real war things will dramatically change.

Things are now quiet again in Wamena, but for how long nobody knows. Do pray for the volatile situation there. The churches are pleading for their people to stay calm and not get involved but of course the mob spirit is contagious. The leaders have asked for a day of prayer and fasting this week. Pray for the church as a whole. Many now have hatred and bitterness in their hearts over what has happened and it is going to take a long time to heal and be forgiven for the wrongs on both sides. Many people are living in refugee camps because they are too scared to go home as many homes were looted.

The missionaries and church folk have been going out to far away villages to buy food for them. The markets and shops were closed. Most of the bridges were torn out so there are no taxis going to the outer areas. Praise the Lord that things are almost back to normal.

For several weeks there have been no planes flying in or out of Wamena as it is still too tense. Then one of the MAF planes was making a normal run to Ninia and he crashed on landing. It would seem the pilot couldn't really concentrate after all the horrors he had witnessed in Wamena and therefore made a mistake on landing. In the midst of this upheaval life went on as usual here in Korupun except for the rumours and speculation and maybe the need to send 200 young men from this area to help in the fighting. I was thankful when that was vetoed. (December 2000)

Jessie retired to Australia soon after this report, but her 'bush telegraph' kept her well informed on developments which she enthusiastically passed on to others.

News from West Papua is good at the moment. Things are quiet. One piece of information is that the government is cracking down on riots and rioters. Anyone carrying a gun, knife or other kind of weapon in the streets is immediately put in jail. Anyone wanting to serve with an overseas army (This comment most likely refers to OPM guerrilla forces operating from across the border in Papua New Guinea) *will automatically lose their citizenship. Strong measures, but very needful at this time. The people still want their freedom, but it would appear that they are now more willing to negotiate, although there are always the hard headed ones who want to go about it with weapons and a 'freedom at any price' attitude. Continue to pray for the pastors and elders that they will keep their priorities straight and their eyes on Jesus instead of material things.*

I was thankful to receive this report of the situation in Wamena: 'There is peace and tranquillity in Wamena again that has been missing since the troubles last year. People are smiling again, schools packed with kids, new businesses opening up and the church has activities that include all the church areas.' (December 2001)

With the rise of radical Islam in Indonesia in the post September 11 world, Jessie was soon alerting her readers to a new fear among many Christians in a more autonomous West Papua.

The government has granted autonomy to the Irian Jaya people, plus some compensation from the mines to help their new government get established. We are not sure how this will work or how much money they will eventually receive. They are also allowed to call the country Papua. We have also been very concerned about information that terrorist training camps have been established in some out of the way places in Irian Jaya. Pray the government will clamp down on them. Pray too for the safety of the pastors and church leaders. They will be the first ones targeted by these groups, just as they were in Ambon. (March 2002)

In spite of all the political unrest and rumours the church quietly continues its teaching and work, but there is an underlying unease knowing that the Laskar Jihad (al Qaeda type) training camps are still in operation in Irian Jaya. The Irianese people have requested the Indonesian Government have them removed but their pleas have fallen on deaf ears and there has been no response. A church in Fak Fak (in the far west or 'bird's head' region) was burnt down and three prominent Papuan leaders have died in suspicious circumstances in the past six months. Pray that the leaders will be able to keep the young people from any unwise retaliation moves that could start a riot when they are provoked by outsiders. (July 2002)

News from Irian Jaya/Papua continues to give us many reasons for concern and prayer regarding the terrorist training camps which have now grown to seven. Apparently when the J.I. (Jemaah Islamiyah, the Indonesian terrorist group behind the Bali bombing and other atrocities) was disbanded in Ambon they moved to Irian. Do pray for the pastors and elders as they know they will be targeted. The Bali bombing has brought this closer to home and shows what they are capable of doing. The Indonesian Government can no longer say they do not exist. (December 2002)

The ongoing problem with the terrorist training camps continues and I have heard that they now have 12 of these camps in Irian. Three of these are close to the PNG border. This is an extract from a concerned PNG newsletter: 'Currently 200 plus men are undergoing terrorism training in a jungle hideout outside Jayapura city. We should not downplay the idea that these terrorists will make plans to infiltrate PNG.' (April 2003)

There have been some sad and difficult situations in the central town of Wamena over the past months when some guns were stolen from the military base there. Certain individuals were immediately targeted and several punished without trial. One man died from the punishment, others beaten and kicked, women raped and houses burnt down for no real reason. It was later established that it was people within the military along with others who had stolen the guns. It would appear that this was a show of strength to intimidate and discourage the people from pushing ahead for their independence. (August 2003)

There is continuing pressure on the missionaries because of the unstable political scene. We have heard that five missionaries with another mission have recently lost their visas. The threat of attacks from the terrorist camps against the local Christian population is a real concern and much prayer is needed for their safety. Although the people in Irian have constantly requested the Indonesian Government remove these camps, they have not done so. On the contrary, thousands more military personnel have moved into the country on one pretext or another. (November 2003)

News from Wesley Dale who has just recently returned from Irian Jaya stated that although things are reasonably calm on the surface, there is still an element of unrest bubbling under the surface. The government elections have not yet been properly completed which is frustrating to the people, plus the fact that new tax laws on homes and land have been implemented for the first time. This has caused much heated discussion among the people and caused instability in some areas. (July 2004)

30. Payback for the postman

They eventually discovered his body and our mail bags hidden beside a log.

Some years ago Elinor and I were in Korupun and the MAF decided that our airstrip needed a major upgrade so we had to close it. One of our male missionaries offered to come in and work on it with the people and manage the work for three weeks. While Chris, the manager, was at Korupun we had no way of getting our mail in and out except by sending a man across the trail to the nearest airstrip which was Sela Valley. When we heard that a plane was scheduled to land in the Sela Valley we would send a man from Korupun to Sela with our mail to go out and he would wait for the plane and bring incoming mail back to us. It was a nine-hour trek across the mountains to Sela.

The airstrip was closed for three months which meant that this same man travelled back and forth as our postman or the 'pony express' to take our mail across the trail to Sela Valley. The trail was very steep and slippery in the wet season. It went over a 10,000 foot mountain which was often cold and wet. Many people died of hypothermia.

One particular day the postman left Korupun in plenty of time to meet the plane the next morning and should have been back by the next after-noon. We waited and waited for him to return but he did not come back that night. We checked with his family in case he was sick and had fallen. They assured us that he had probably stopped at one of the villages or had gone the long way round to visit some relatives and told us not to worry for a couple more days.

The next day when he did not return we again enquired among the local people if they had heard any word of him from the other direction. His relatives decided to send some of his friends along the trail to see if he had had an accident. When they didn't find any sign of him or his net bag on the trail, they decided that some foul play had happened. Normally, when someone is ill or caught on the high mountain and become chilled, they will creep off the main path into a crevice or a log or somewhere to keep warm. They would leave something to alert people on the main path that they are nearby.

Again they did not find anything to alert them to his whereabouts. They came back and called a church meeting and asked all the churches in the valley to pray all night so that God would show them where he was or what was happening to him. Time was against them as he could die or clues could be lost regarding what had happened to him. After praying all night they went home and slept. Three different men from three different villages had the same dream of a certain part of the trail that he would have taken. They sent out search parties two by two along this particular stretch of the trail and into the dense bushes on either side. They eventually discovered his body and our mail bags hidden beside a log. This was in a part of the trail which the men had seen in their dream. They brought him home for a cremation and then decided to track down those who had been the perpetrators of the crime.

They are very clever at finding clues and within a day they knew exactly who had done it and why. They went across to Sela Valley to talk to the relatives of these people whom they were quite sure had killed him. They discovered that there had been some money put in the bag for someone in Korupun. These men had heard that there was money. They also had a grievance against the postman's family because one of their women had been taken as a wife by someone in Korupun and they had not completed the marriage dowry payments of pigs and other items. They felt justified in killing him as payment for non-payment of the marriage dowry by the post-man's relatives. The 'detectives' from Korupun then talked to many people in the Sela Valley and discovered that the men they were looking for had absconded to the south and had hidden in the lowlands.

A group of people from Korupun decided to track the two men down and within three to four days found the two men and brought them back to be tried by the village chief. They brought them across the trail from Sela with much shouting and jubilation. They sat the men in the middle of the airstrip and danced around them shouting and singing their cannibal songs. After pretending to shoot them with arrows and spitting on them and shouting curses the people decided to tie them up and take them to Wamena to put them in jail. As many of the people were Christians they did not want to kill them. The relatives of these men very hurriedly gathered up some pigs in payment for the death of the postman. This was the usual manner of payback if someone is killed. They brought the pigs to Korupun travelling through the night and were there by the following morning. The relatives of the postman killed and ate the pigs that had been brought over as payment for the death of the postman.

After much deliberation the government official in Korupun decided to take them out to Wamena, starting the following day – this took 10 days walk. The next night several of the prisoners' relatives crept into the house where the men were kept and let them go free. As the relatives had eaten the peace-meal of pigs they decided to let the two men go and not pursue them. We did hear rumours afterwards that they had planned to push the two men over the cliff on the way to Wamena. This would have added fuel to the fire for further payback. Both sides were appeased with the decision they had made.

31. Goodbye to the highlands

I have been able to go to all the main areas to say goodbye.

It was a busy time for Jessie as she embarked on a last tour of the highlands, dropping in on the familiar towns and villages to farewell her many friends and colleagues.

It is hard to believe that my time here has almost come to an end after 34 years living and working here amongst the Dani and Kimyal people. It has been a privilege to see God at work and witness His miracles amongst these stone-age warriors. God has changed these people from the inside out whereas civilisation just changes them on the outside and leaves the unchanged savage inside. It was rather an emotional time....

Last week I went to Sela Valley for a new clinic opening. I stayed several days and they had a farewell feast for me as well. It was fun to be back again in my little house over there, but not so funny when a little lizard fell off the ceiling in fright and dropped down my neck. It was good to have time to say goodbye to everyone. I will be leaving here at the end of December and this will be a closure of a chapter of my life but a new beginning of something else. I will attend the Field Conference in January and say goodbye to all my colleagues and then head homewards. (December 2000)

My last month in Irian was filled to capacity with many special occasions. The graduation of the last group of clinic workers changed from a small family feast to a large farewell occasion for me as well as the graduation feast for the trainees. Because there were so many wanting to attend it was by invitation only. Even so they killed 31 pigs with lots of rabbits and chickens. The place was buzzing with excitement. They had the ceremony outside as the church was too small to hold the crowd. The graduates received their diplomas and then there were speeches and farewell speeches. Pastor Siud said: 'God sent Jessie here when she was young and her hair was brown and now her hair is white and she is all shrivelled up.' It's nice to have truthful friends isn't it? He also asked me to thank the Christian people in Australia who had prayed for them in the past to continue to do the same in future, especially in this politically tense and uncertain time.

I had quite a number of visitors in early December which was great. I stayed in Korupun for Christmas and had the elders and clinic workers in for a special Christmas meal. I then began packing and sorting of many things I had had for 30 years, distributing the contents to those who wanted or needed them. I had hoped to get it all done quickly the week after Christmas but when the people realised that I would be leaving in a week they all came to visit me and say farewell. Some came to cry, others to say goodbye, some to give me a hug and a prayer and others just sat and sat and didn't want to go home. Yet others came from distant villages and said: 'I have walked three days to see your face once more.' It was a very emotional time, time consuming, and not at all easy.

I sent my little dog out to Wamena to a family who were happy to care for her properly. In the process of trying to get her in the 'pod' of the plane she was very frightened and bit me through the sack we had put her in to travel out to Wamena. That didn't help me to get on with my packing with a bandaged hand, plus the hydro going off for two nights and therefore no electricity.

Because of the uncertainty of the political situation it was decided to change the venue of our annual conference from the cooler highlands to the hot coastal area of Sentani. I was able to be part of the conference for several days before departure. Most of my colleagues were there at the airport to see me off which was very special. I was very thankful to the

Lord that my trip home was uneventful although we had several hiccoughs at Sentani when we realised that my passport had not been put into the immigration for an 'exit only', meaning that I would not be returning and couldn't get out of the country. Dave made a special trip to Jayapura that night especially to get it cleared. (March 2001)

32. Like the prodigal son

When I left Irian the people said they hoped to have the dedication of the New Testament in two years' time and that they wanted me to come back for the occasion. Then they qualified the statement by saying if it wasn't done in two years I'd be dead!!! To them I am already as old as Methuselah and my time is running out. (September 2001)

Jessie maintained a lifelong interest in West Papua, staying in contact with old friends and colleagues and keeping abreast of developments there. When the chance came to return for a visit she jumped at it with the same enthusiasm that first brought her to the highlands.

Brian Billing, our World Team director for Australia asked if I would be willing to return to Papua for a month to accompany Nicole, a uni student who feels called to work there, and would like to do a mission awareness trip to the area. As you can imagine I was happy to fall in with the plans to leave in late January. We would value your prayer for safety as we travel through Indonesia. (November 2004)

The past month could be termed a nostalgic walk down memory lane. After the night flight we arrived very weary to a very hot, humid Sentani, where we were met by a missionary colleague, Rosanna, who kindly transported us to where we were to stay the next couple of days. Sentani and Jayapura have expanded. Lots of new stores. Others had been burnt down in the riots of several years ago and the new stores built. A new KFC had recently opened and we patronised it by having KFC chicken with rice Irian style.

Flying out of Sentani with Regions Wings we landed in Taiyeve in the steamy Lakes Plains where I had worked for a year and trained some clinic workers before I moved to Korupun. It was good to catch up with one of them. We enjoyed a canoe trip on the river to cool off and have a swim. We were glad the crocs were sleeping while we were in the water. We then flew to Wamena in the mountains to stay with Sue Trenier. She is the medical coordinator for the Eastern Highlands area and oversees Korupun from a distance. The cool air was very refreshing. There are now quite a few street children in Wamena. Some have come hoping for work and bored with village life, others have dropped out of school for one reason or another and have not gone home and have nowhere to live. In spite of there being a government hospital in the town the little clinic run by the church is always busy because the patients say the clinic workers care about them and will pray with them. With Papua now being divided into three provinces a lot of changes are forecast. Some changes are good and others not so good.

After two busy days we climbed into the Heli Mission helicopter and flew to Tokuni for four days. The Martin family live there in the middle of the steamy jungle. Allyson and Kevin are learning the language and hoping to reduce it into writing so they can translate the scriptures. It was back to being under a mosquito net at nights and washing and bathing in the river each afternoon. I worked with the two clinic workers teaching them how to suture on a lemon and also how to reduce and splint a fractured limb. Allyson and Kevin also wanted to know how to take a blood pressure reading and put in an intravenous if the need arose. Up and away again as the helicopter took us to Obukain, which is half-an-hour away to the east, to stay with the Johnson family for six days at their jungle outpost. Nicole taught school to the three Johnson children each morning while I worked with the clinic worker I had trained some years ago and taught him and the pastor about some of the new medications and also how to reduce and splint a fracture.

We arrived back in Wamena late in the afternoon before heading to Korupun at the crack of dawn. The weather was good and we were off. We were greeted like the prodigal son. Hugs all round. Chucked under the chin and clasped to more manly chests than I can remember in one day and cried over as if I had returned from the dead. Everyone was so pleased to see us. The house was constantly full of people coming and greeting us. Sabil, the head clinic worker, came as often as he could because he said 'you are only here for one week and I want to see your face to remember it well.'

The next morning we flew to Deibula. It is a four-day trek, but 15 minutes by heli, to be part of the dedication of a new clinic. Great excitement with a pig feast, speeches and welcome. Again I was hugged and cried over by all the clinic workers who had come for the special occasion. I was given a live pig. After a couple of hours of eating their special delicacies the heli manoeuvred through the fog to return to Korupun. At church (that Sunday) they asked me the question: 'Now you are here why can't you stay?' The fact that I was getting old was not a viable excuse to them, as they said I looked very healthy. It is always a good feeling to be wanted but they need to be independent and trust the Lord for their needs and for wisdom. It was the plan to work my way out of a job. (March 2005)

Jessie wasn't yet finished with West Papua. She would make one more visit to her beloved Korupun.

After months of delay, uncertainty and change of plans and dates, it seems likely that the dedication of the Kimyal New Testament will at last come to fruition in February 2010. Rosa went to Java in October to finalise all the finer details of the formatting and layout for the printing. The Kimyals of course are very excited and have grandiose ideas for that special day. They have invited all the former missionaries who have worked in the area over the years. It will include Phyliss Masters, Rosa and Orin Kidd, Elinor Young, Judy and Bruce McLeay and me. I am planning to go with a long-time friend – Jessie Legge. I believe life in Irian Jaya/Papua has changed dramatically since I was there a couple of years ago. (December 2009)

The New Testament dedication held in West Papua during March, was a trip down memory lane for those who had worked in Korupun over the past 40 years. My friend Jessie Legge and I had an uneventful trip to Sentani. We were welcomed by a group of Kimyal students studying at the university there. They insisted on taking us out for a meal where they paid the bill!!! After several days of waiting to get our 'permission to travel' we flew to Wamena and spent a couple of days with my Irish friend and former colleague Sue Trenier and saw her work amongst the AIDS and TB patients. We parted from Wamena courtesy of MAF at 5.30 am on a very misty day headed for Korupun.

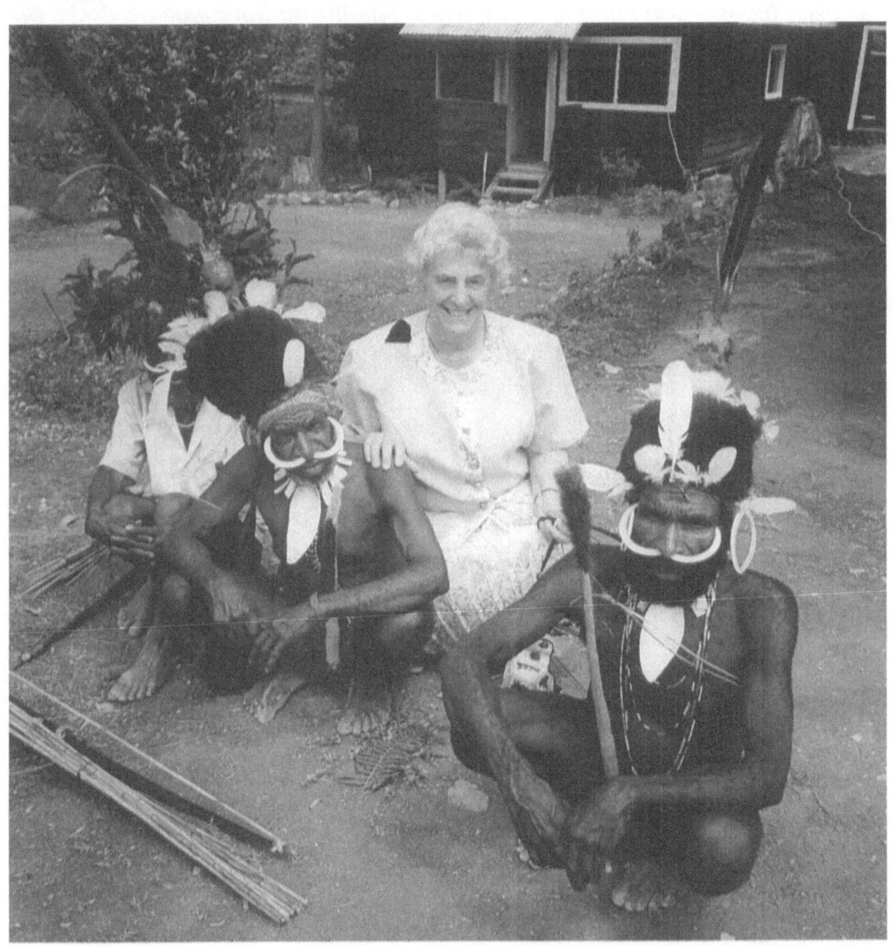

We were welcomed by a huge crowd of excited people. They greeted us with a gift of a necklace of local beads and many hugs. The local band was playing as the people sang, chanted and danced around us, many decked out in their finery of feathers, large net bags and painted faces. They had been dancing for days and their enthusiasm was infectious. The rugged mountains, swirling mists, creeping fog and thundering rains had not changed, but many of our Kimyal friends now had grey hair as did most of the attending missionaries.

The week of the dedication was a fulfilment of all their hopes and dreams to read the Word of God in their own language in one book. Praise God he has used his Word to change many lives. The initial language analysis, alphabet and some translation was accomplished by Elinor, until she had to return home due to health reasons. The Lord challenged Rosa Kidd to take up the unfinished task. She felt very inadequate but began the translation before she too had to return home due to family and health reasons. Rosa continued to work from home in conjunction with two National translators. She returned to the field for two months every two years. Now, after 15 years of perseverance, the New Testament is completed.

Three days before the dedication a MAF plane brought in the boxes of New Testaments. The air was charged with emotion as the first box was given to the pastors and elders. Many were weeping. Pastor Siud prayed and thanked God for this very special day when they would have the Word of God in their own language under one cover. He said he felt like Simeon when he held the baby Jesus in his arms and he could see the fulfilment of the prophecy of the Messiah. The box was given to the old people who had prayed for this day, and was then passed onto the young people adjured to read God's Word to lead them in the way of righteousness.

The day of the dedication began with excitement mounting to fever pitch when the people were woken to start making fires, killing over 100 pigs and chickens and preparing the vegetables etc. Organised chaos like an ant hill. Everyone knows their duties and does it. The vice-governor and his party duly arrived and the celebrations began with prayer and praise sung by the school children from different villages. Many people dressed as warriors re-enacted the coming of the first missionaries and how they had planned to put them into the spirit house, hang them up and kill them. Instead the men gave out gifts of salt and peanuts which they received. Salt being a precious commodity they decided not to kill them. Many speeches followed. After the formality of cutting the ribbon Phyliss Masters opened the packages of New Testaments. She gave the first copy to Pastor Siud which caused great rejoicing from the people. Siud thanked the missionaries for coming and bringing them God's Word which has changed their lives. (June 2010)

In this newsletter Jessie also recounted a general reflection made by several of the missionaries that the current (third) generation of Kimyal Christians didn't *know the darkness, the wars, the cannibalism, the sickness, the deaths and the very bad earthquakes of the 70's and 80's* which had coincided with the original conversions of Kimyal Christians. How quickly time had moved on in the remotest highland areas.

During my recent trip to West Papua it was very special to be part of the enthusiasm of the people to own and read the New Testament in their own language. Each Christmas they would re-enact the Nativity story with a live black baby as Jesus and black faced angels in their white robes. It was a day of celebration. So sad to see the real Christmas slipping into oblivion here (in Australia). Once the dedication of the New Testament and celebrations at Korupun were over, Phyliss Masters, Jessie Legge and myself headed for Dani Karubaga where I had begun my missionary career in 1966. Phyliss had returned there after Phil was killed in 1968 and we had worked there with the Karubaga staff, Phyliss in the medical accommodation section and later in the women's ministry and me in the hospital and clinic work. As we landed on the new, enlarged asphalted airstrip I wondered how many people would remember me after 20 years absence whilst I worked in Korupun. No need to worry that I was forgotten as we were mobbed by people as soon as we stepped off the plane. It took us two hours to work our way to the house as there was a line of people all wanting to be greeted, hugged and hands shaken. A constant refrain to me was: 'I thought you had died' but they were glad to see me in the flesh.

We stayed in the doctor's old house which was quite comfortable except for some uninvited guests we found in the house in the shape of rats, bedbugs, mosquitoes and cockroaches. The people immediately set to work preparing a big pig feast in our front garden. They asked Phyliss to share a ministry with the women and asked me to give some lessons on AIDS which we were happy to do. We were overwhelmed by gifts of veggies, fruit, net bags and meat. I was astonished when an old lady brought me a net bag to say thank-you for saving her husband's life some 25 years previously. Many others brought gifts for the help I had given to their babies all those years ago which I had long since forgotten about. It was a time of reminiscing with them over those early years and putting older faces with grey hair to the people we had known. Sadness for the ones missing from the ranks. We wandered around the city which had grown up since we had left and wondered at the changes. They even had vehicles that travel over the dangerous roads and bridges to bring in supplies from Wamena for the ever growing population of people from other islands - military, police, school teachers, even a bank and mosque. Times have changed and the people are facing many choices and temptations. We need to pray for them. (December 2010)

It was the last time Jessie visited West Papua, though her long-time friend and colleague Sabil made one last effort to encourage Jessie to return when he asked 'are you sure you don't want to come back here to live? I would make sure we would have plenty of wood for your funeral!'

The Kimyal do not bury their dead and the family provides wood for their cremation. Jessie said he must have been thinking she would need a fair bit of wood.

33. Back home - the later years

Once more I am surrounded by boxes and suitcases needing to be unpacked and sorted. This time, in Australia, I go through an accumulation of things stored in my garage over a number of years, plus the suitcases of sentimental things I brought home from Irian Jaya.

When Jessie retired from the field she returned to Melbourne, though she continued to travel within Australia sharing information about World Team and West Papua and continued distributing her prayer letters.

On my way home I took the opportunity of stopping off at Darwin to visit a niece, then on to Sydney to stay with my sister Thelma. Then on to Melbourne and the unpacking! I will need your prayer as I try to get settled in this 'foreign land'. There are so many things I need to learn about shopping and running a household here. Huge supermarkets are a little daunting with all the choice and advertising. Rather different to sending in an order form to our agents in Jayapura and then being surprised at what comes three months later on the plane. (March 2001)

Do you realise that it is now 35 years that you have been receiving my prayer letters and have been part of my team of prayer warriors. I have greatly appreciated the faithfulness and expertise of my sister Vera and brother-in-law Ken, who have faithfully sent out my prayer letters over the years. Many, many hours of work. Now it is my turn to do more than just write and send it off. (September 2001)

Not surprisingly it took some time to make the transition from Jessie's busy village life to semi-retirement in Melbourne.

They tell me it will take five to 10 years before I really feel 'at home' here in Australia socially and emotionally. There have been so many changes to get used to; it takes time to adjust to them all. Of course Irian Jaya is never far away from my thoughts most days and I often wonder how they are coping. (September 2001)

Retirement also brought new opportunities. Jessie was asked to attend a study school in Canada involving missionaries from around the world. She jumped at the chance to spend two months in Canada and the United States.

It was a time of learning new concepts, mind stretching, fun and fellowship as we all worked together in teams. Following the month in Canada I was excited to visit many old friends in the U.S.A. who had lived and worked in Irian Jaya years ago. It was good to reminisce of days gone by. (September 2001)

In 2001 Jessie enjoyed just the third Christmas she had spent in Australia in 35 years. She began her new job as prayer coordinator for World Team *to link people up in a huge prayer chain in Australia. I am not too sure as to the best way to go about getting it all together. Another first for me and another challenge to trust the Lord in a new way.* (December 2001)

She continued to travel with her work, connecting with family, friends and supporters around Australia, and still keen to test herself physically with new challenges.

When I was in Sydney my sister Thelma gave me a ticket to do 'the bridge climb' for my birthday. This is one of the newest tourist attractions in Sydney. We climbed the span of the Sydney Harbour Bridge right up to the flags. (December 2001)

We have had an unexpected sadness in our family when my sister Vera suddenly passed away in October after an 18 months battle with leukaemia. We are thankful that she was spared a long, debilitating illness, although it was very hard for us having her go so unexpectedly. But death is not the end for those of us who have trusted Jesus — it is just a new beginning. (December 2001).

Jessie's brother-in-law Ken passed away in August the following-year after a short illness with a brain tumour. *Vera and Ken both gone within a year is not what we anticipated.* (December 2002)

Whoever said to me that 'life must be boring for you now that you have retired' should have been with me over the past three months. It has certainly been packed with new experiences. During February and March I accompanied Phyllis Masters as she travelled and spoke in many different venues in Tasmania, Victoria and New South Wales. It was good to catch up with some of you on our travels. Phyllis has a very special message to give. We met up with many relatives and friends of Stan Dale on our travels. Many of them prayed for Phyllis over the years so it was good for them to meet face to face. (April 2003)

Last week I got a surprise when I opened up the computer to find two messages in the Kimyal language there for me. The clinic workers had written letters and given them to Sue Trenier to send to me through the email. One from Sabil asking for prayer as they are finding it harder to get the medications they need if they have an epidemic. He mentioned that 18 had died from amoebic dysentery because of the lack of the right drugs.

Some exciting news to hand is that I have been chosen to go as a delegate to the World Team Conference in Hungary in March. It will be my first trip to Europe. I hope to meet up with many co-workers from past years. (November 2003)

My trip to Europe to visit so many old friends was fantastic and I enjoyed every minute of it. People were so kind and helpful everywhere I went. They all killed the 'fatted calf' and took me to all their favourite places.

She visited many places including Holland, Switzerland, France, Germany, Italy and Great Britain. In London she did the usual tourist things — visiting the Australian War Memorial in Hyde Park, watching the changing of the guard at Buckingham Palace and wandering around Windsor Castle, the Tower Bridge and the Tower of London.

It was very special to meet up with my friend Sue Trenier who is still working in Irian Jaya but was on furlough in the UK. She was leaving to return to Papua in three days' time. We sat and ate waffles and ice-cream in Covent Garden and talked and talked. There couldn't have been a vaster contrast as our ways separated to leave me in London and her back to the wilds of Irian Jaya. (July 2004)

After a hurried trip to Cambridge and Keswick in the Lake District Jessie visited Scotland, reconnecting with Jack Leng, one of her first colleagues when she arrived in Karubaga.

Jack was the Doctor who operated on Stan Dale in 1966 which was my introduction to life in the Karubaga Hospital. They took me the length and breadth of Scotland in a whirlwind visit to Aberdeen, Edinburgh Castle, Holyrood Palace, walked on the shores of Loch Lomond, drove along the road the Romans built, walked on Hadrian's Wall, ate and enjoyed all kinds of Scottish delicacies. In fact I was spoilt rotten but enjoyed it all. (July 2004)

Jessie called the trip her *trip of a lifetime*, stopping off in the United States on her journey home to visit Rosa and Orin Kidd whom she worked with in Korupun. Back in Australia, the turning of the years was continuing to take its toll on her family.

Another sad event that happened in our family ranks is the loss of our eldest sister, Olive, five months ago. She had been unwell for 18 months with different problems and passed away three weeks after I returned from my trip overseas. I was thankful to be at home at the time. Coming at the tail end of a large family it suddenly happens that as I get older, the ones up ahead are also clocking up the years. I am thankful to be keeping well at present. (November 2004)

But the good health didn't last.

Over recent months I have been seeing a haematologist because my blood had some strange things floating around in it. The final diagnosis last week was that I have a type of leukaemia. At the present time I am stable and I do not need any kind of chemotherapy or medications. My own doctor will continue to monitor my blood levels and he will be made aware if there is any need for medication or chemotherapy later on. As you can imagine this has come as a shock. (June 2008)

I had an appointment to see the haematologist specialist in December. He was surprised and pleased with my blood results as it had not changed from the previous visit. Because it is stable he has not given me any medication and doesn't want to see me for six months. What a wonderful Christmas present. Over these uncertain days the Lord has encouraged me from Isaiah 41; 10. Do not fear, for I am with you, do not be dismayed, for I am your God, I will strengthen you and help you. I will uphold you with my righteous hand. (December 2008/January 2009)

My elder brother Jim passed away in October. He had been failing in health for some time and had been in respite care for one month when he had a massive heart attack and didn't linger. A happy release for him but a break in the chain of memories for the rest of us. (December 2009)

It is amazing how life can change in a few short hours or weeks. Just before Christmas my oncologist was concerned about my blood reports and suggested that I have a bone marrow biopsy to get a clearer picture of how things were progressing. The result was not favourable. He found that I had changed from a low grade leukaemia to an acute myeloid leukaemia which is far more aggressive. I was given the options of different types of chemotherapy or no treatment with six months to live. I had to make a decision. After much prayer I went to see the professor and before I could give him my answer he said: 'I have heard that there is a drug trial for your type of leukaemia starting at the Alfred Hospital. I think it would suit you better as the chemo is reduced and the new tablets have minimal side-affects.' I am now a regular visitor to the Alfred Hospital drug trial most mornings, but that is a long commitment for the next six months as I am not allowed to drive.

Jessie suffered some bad side-effects from the drugs, lost 10 kilograms and spent 10 days in an isolation ward suffering from septicaemia.

I don't remember much of the following 10 days but I am very grateful to the three teams of doctors who discovered, isolated and treated the two bugs in my system. Because I was very shaky on my legs because of the length of time spent in bed and the loss of muscle tone I had to learn how to walk again. It was decided to send me to a rehabilitation hospital for 10 days. I have been so grateful to family and friends who have been so helpful since I came home by staying overnights, cooking meals, cleaning the house and making it easier for me to stay in my own home. After being independent for so long it is hard to stay put and let others do it....When I went back to my first review with the doctor at the trial clinic he was amazed when he read my blood results and couldn't believe that they were so good. He said to me, you have had such a bad reaction to the drug, been put through the mangle and we nearly lost you, but your blood levels are better than they were three months ago. I replied that I had a lot of people praying for me. (June 2011)

34. The last word

I hesitantly stepped onto Indonesian soil, feeling very inadequate, and very naïve about the situation to which I was headed. Let's take a walk down memory lane as we remember God's goodness and faithfulness over the years.

On 14 May 1991 Jessie clocked up 25 years' service in West Papua. In her regular update to friends and supporters at the time, she reflected on these years. Her words touch on the adventures, the triumphs, the struggles and the joys she found in the mountains, particularly among her Kimyal friends. While another 10 years of missionary service still lay ahead of her at the time she made these jottings, I found no other writing that more succinctly summed up the driving forces in her life, her work and her faith – a faith that sustained her through many difficult times, and comforted her in her last days.

So many changes have come and gone in those years. Even the name of the country changed three times, but God has not changed. He remains faithful. We have seen truly amazing things happen in the lives of those stone-age people, many who had never seen a white man, let alone white woman in those days. Our God is truly the God of the impossible, as we have seen hardened killers, cannibals and witch doctors change dramatically as they turned from spirit worship to faith in what Jesus had done for them. He took away the very fear of demons, gave them hope for the future, and freedom from fear of death.

Thirteen years were spent running the hospital and the baby clinic at Karubaga for the Dani people. It was a very busy and demanding program. One of my first cases after I had been there just 10 days, was to nurse Stan Dale after he had been shot the first time. Responsibilities varied, as personnel changed, and different slots needed to be filled. These ranged from hospital supervisor, airport manager and radio coordinator, to buying 2000 pounds of vegies each week, to be transported to Sentani for the missionaries there, to taking a women's and children's Bible class, training clinic workers, running the station generator and caring for the welfare of the cows. When the hospital was closed because we couldn't get a visa for a new doctor I spent a year at Taiyeve in the northern lowlands relieving the nurse there so she could go on furlough. Very different in the hot swamps instead of the cool mountains. I became a 'flying nurse' as I accompanied the pilots to many of the villages scattered throughout the swamps. This was a very different and challenging program, but once again the Lord was there beside me to encourage and help. Many of the people had never seen a white woman so I came in for my share of hair pulling and pinching to see if the white would come off. Diagnosing and giving advice over the radio to teachers on these lonely outposts was a big responsibility.

The last 11 years at Korupun amongst the pygmy cannibals has been a special experience. Exciting to see the changes come into so many lives as they turned their backs on appeasing the evil spirits and handed their lives to the Lord. It has been encouraging to see the clinic workers start from the grass roots level to taking on the responsibilities for the wellbeing of their people, both spiritual and physical, as they work alongside the evangelist or pastor. It has been thrilling to hear their stories of how often the Lord has answered their prayers for different patients, and also giving wisdom when they needed it.

Great to see the literacy programme in which I was involved for some time, now taken over by a very competent local man whom the Lord is using to reach many people as he teaches a Bible class before literacy begins. The

Bible school is now running efficiently on its own with National teachers. The students are very keen to get any new scripture portions that Elinor translates for them. Seeing the church outgrow its buildings, and having to rebuild, and them become concerned for others outside of their regions who have not heard the Gospel has been a real encouragement. Seeing God at work in the hearts and lives of the people is a real privilege. Pray for the church that it will continue to grow in the knowledge of the Lord.

Through all these different tasks and changes the Lord has been so faithful. When I have been discouraged, He has encouraged; when I have been exasperated, He has given me patience; when I have been angry, He has given me love; when I have been so weary, He has given me wisdom. I praise and thank the Lord for his forgiveness, caring and constant love over these years. As he promised when I came to Irian Jaya He has remained the same, the God of the impossible. And you, my faithful prayer and financial supporters, have been a large part of the Lord's program up here. I could never have survived without your constant prayer concern, love and financial help. We are workers together - His church in the hearts and lives of the people of Irian Jaya. Thank you for your faithfulness, please continue to pray that the Lord will be central in our work, and that His name will be glorified throughout these mountains.

It was, and remains, a fitting epitaph to Jessie's life's work.

Her trials, tribulations, triumphs, humour and optimism were always shared with her small army of supporters in Australia, both family and friends, and their support came in many ways – financial, spiritual, and towards the end, as ill-health sapped her physical strength and robbed her of much of her prized independence - through daily care and attention. Some of these special long-term friends, Pam and Jim Sterrey, Marlene Davey and Wendy Crew, and of course as always, her surviving sisters, Pam, Jean and Thelma, gave practical assistance and comfort throughout Jessie's battle with the leukaemia that would eventually claim her life.

Despite the onset of this debilitating illness, Jessie was determined to remain independent, albeit it with considerable assistance from family and friends. She was admitted to the Alfred Hospital for the last time on Sunday

4 May 2014. It had been clear Jessie's health was deteriorating. Thelma remembers that just a few weeks before Jess entered hospital:

'I had sensed Jess was not really coping and came down (from her home at Woy Woy north of Sydney) for two weeks, I was reluctant to go home and of course it was only about a week before I was back to help arrange the funeral.'

Jessie's sister Pam who lived nearby was with her at the end. Pam provided this account of Jessie's last days:

'In the weeks preceding her passing, Jess had been managing at home with some help – but becoming more frail - but being Jess, was still up and around. On Friday 2 May I had taken her for a quick shop and then returned home for a nice lunch together. She had her usual snooze in her chair after lunch – but seemed quite ok – as usual. Then on Saturday she called friends to ask if they could come and do a small gardening job for her. They arrived, completed the job and enjoyed a lovely afternoon tea and chat. That Sunday, friends came to visit at 12 noon and found her still in bed with a high fever. They called the ambulance and she was immediately transferred to The Alfred where she had been undergoing her treatment. As soon as the staff who had been treating Jessie learnt she was in the hospital, they convinced the authorities to transfer Jessie upstairs from ICU into their care. As they said: 'Jess wouldn't like it down there, it's too noisy!!' So, like an old friend, Jess remained in the care of the staff who had been treating her for the past two years. Our sister Jean, her daughter Judy and I spent Sunday and Monday afternoon and evenings with Jess and although she was under heavy medication, she occasionally responded by opening her eyes and/or giving a slight smile when we stroked or kissed her – but was very peaceful.

On Tuesday 6 May Jean, Judy and I visited around noon. Jess was in a deep, peaceful sleep but there was no response to our overtures. We decided to leave at 3pm and return later in the day/evening. As we were getting settled into Judy's car at the hospital, I had this overwhelming feeling that I HAD to stay. I couldn't go. Jean and Judy left intending to return later. I went back in to be with Jess. Shortly after, Danny Hunt, Jess's Pastor arrived for a visit. Danny and I were sitting beside Jess's bed talking quietly, when I suddenly realised that she wasn't breathing. She had just slipped away – so peacefully – and, as you would expect from Jess, without fuss!!'

Officiating at Jessie's memorial service on 14 May 2014 Pastor Hunt said: 'If a church is allowed to have heroes, Jessie is one of our heroes.'

Shortly before the service a final message came by email from the Kimyals thanking Jessie for coming to them. It shall be our last word on Jessie's wonderful life:

'You have been completed, Goodbye…….'

Acknowledgements

I hope Jessie's *House of Needles* is close to the book Jessie might have written had her hectic life and, in her last years, failing health permitted her to do so. Though I never knew Jessie personally I feel I have come to know her through her writings which form the core of this memoir, and the personal insights of the many people who wanted Jessie's story told, particularly her sister Thelma and brother-in-law Jim Minto, and other surviving siblings Jean, Pamela and Gordon who entrusted me with the telling.

We have also been assisted by Jessie's missionary colleagues and friends who have shared their memories and observations. Most particularly I want to thank Dr Les Henson and his wife Wapke, long time colleagues and friends of Jessie in both West Papua and later in Melbourne where Les now teaches and supervises postgraduate students in missiology. Their intimate knowledge of West Papua, missions and local Papuan culture, history and belief systems has been invaluable in ensuring both accuracy and historical context and I greatly appreciate their efforts and support. I also thank Don Richardson for writing the foreword and for his other positive feedback in helping ensure the authenticity of the text.

My role was to edit, collate, provide context and weave Jessie's words into a narrative that accurately captured the flavour of her life and times in missionary service in West Papua, and share excerpts from her remarkable life, experiences and insights with others. While Jessie's words have been edited for style, consistency, accuracy and clarity, I have endeavoured to retain Jessie's authentic voice and the context in which her words were written.

I have read and researched widely to fill in the background to Jessie's original words however five books have been particularly instructive and small extracts of all five are quoted in the text. The full references for these works are:

Decker, John with Lois Neeley 1992, *Torches of Joy*, YWAM Publishing, Seattle.

Reeson, Margaret 1972, *Torn Between Two Worlds*, Kristen Pres, Madang PNG.

Richardson, Don 2005, *Peace Child*, 4th Edition, Regal, California, U.S.A.

Richardson, Don 2014, *Lords of the Earth*, Bethany House edition, Minneapolis, Minnesota

Wick, Dr Robert S. 1990, *God's Invasion*, Buena Book Services a division of Christian Publications, Camp Hill, Pennsylvania.

The quotations at the front of this book are edited excerpts from a 2010 interview with Jessie Williamson broadcast in: *'The Kimyal Tribe: The Gospel History'* (World Team 2013).

I would also like to give special thanks to my wife Sally whose wise counsel, editing, technical and design skills contributed so much in converting a draft manuscript into this final published form.

I hope you have enjoyed getting to know Jessie. I certainly have.

John Algate